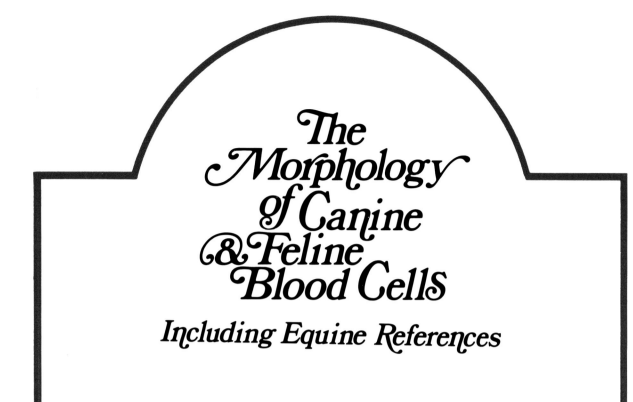

The Morphology of Canine & Feline Blood Cells

Including Equine References

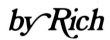

by Rich

By Lon J. Rich, D.V.M., Ph.D.
Colorado State University
College of Veterinary Medicine
and Biomedical Sciences
Department of Clinical Sciences
Ft. Collins, Colorado

RALSTON PURINA COMPANY: Checkerboard Square, St. Louis, Missouri 63188

Form GP 2880B   76002   Printed in U.S.A.

Foreword

This is the first reprinting of Dr. Rich's monograph on canine and feline hematology. It was originally printed in 1974. Its praise and popularity by the veterinary profession has met and exceeded our greatest expectations.

You will find this second edition includes an update on the table of Normal Blood Values for Dogs and Cats, with the addition of values for the geriatric pet. Blood samples for these studies were collected at the Purina Pet Care Center, Gray Summit, Missouri.

We trust these color prints of normal and pathologic cells will be of special assistance in your practice. "The Morphology of Canine & Feline Blood Cells," and many other Purina veterinary and client aids, are testimony to the importance of the small animal practitioner in today's society. These aids are an outgrowth of the indepth research that stands behind all Purina pet foods.

The Professional Marketing Services Department of the Ralston Purina Company is pleased to present this canine and feline reference as still another service in support of the veterinary profession's quest to provide better health for the pet population.

T. B. Follis, DVM, PhD
Manager, Veterinary Services
Professional Marketing Services Dept.

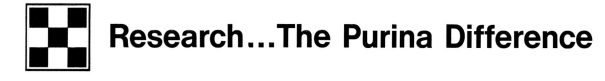

Research...The Purina Difference

Contents

Introduction

The first comprehensive veterinary hematology book was published by Dr. O. W. Schalm in 1961. Since that time there has been an upsurge of interest in veterinary hematology. Veterinarians are performing complete blood counts (CBC's) in their own offices as well as sending large numbers of blood samples to diagnostic laboratories for evaluation. Yet there is no complete animal morphology book that the veterinarian or technician can refer to for cell identification. Pathologic abnormalities are described in specific papers but are generally unavailable for quick reference. The purpose of this monograph is to provide readily accessible photographs and simple descriptions of various blood cells encountered in both normal and selected abnormal disease conditions. The first part of this monograph is concerned with normal peripheral blood and bone marrow morphology; the last part deals with morphologic abnormalities.

Examination of blood cells, when correlated with the case history and physical examination, may provide information relative to (1) the definitive diagnosis in a few instances, (2) alternate diagnoses, (3) prognosis of a particular case and (4) effectiveness of treatment. The use of blood morphology to make a definitive diagnosis or to provide alternate diagnoses will be emphasized by using illustrative cases.

All slides used in this preparation were made from fresh blood without anticoagulant. These were stained with Wright's stain (Appendix I) and photographed with the Zeiss Photomicroscope using Kodak photomicrography color film 2483. This film was selected because of its high color saturation and definition at some expense of accurate reproduction of red color. Figures 1 and 2 were photographed initially with Kodacolor X, through the use of increased amplitude with Normarski differential interference optics, a method devised by David and Williamson. The cells were cut out, mounted and then copied with Kodak photomicrography film.

I. Normal Bone Marrow and Blood Cytology

NOMENCLATURE

The classification of blood cells (Table 1) generally follows that recommended by the Committee for Clarification of the Nomenclature of Cells and Diseases of the Blood and Blood-Forming Organs.

CELL MORPHOLOGY— GENERAL CONCEPTS

Most Cells, if not all, that appear in peripheral blood have their origin from the bone marrow "stem cell." The morphology of this "stem cell" is in disagreement among hematologists, but many believe that it is morphologically indistinguishable from the small lymphocyte found in the bone marrow. This bone marrow small lymphocyte is thus totipotent, giving rise to erythrocytes, leukocytes, monocytes, lymphocytes, plasma cells *and* platelets (Table 1). Since cells in the peripheral blood come from the bone marrow, it is appropriate to study the normal maturation sequence of each cell type as it appears in the bone marrow.

MATURATION SEQUENCE

As cells develop their morphology changes. These morphologic alterations occur gradually, hence many cells are in transition from one named cell type to another. By convention, cells in transition are classified towards the more differentiated cell type. Thus, if there is a question whether a cell is a rubricyte or a metarubricyte, call it the latter.

Immature cells are generally larger and become smaller as they mature. The nuclei of the immature cells are relatively large in relation to the amount of cytoplasm and become smaller with maturity. In immature cells, the chromatin of the nucleus is delicate, fine and reticulated. As the cell matures the chromatin becomes coarse, clumped and compact. Nucleoli are found in the nucleus of immature cells; they vary in size and number but are generally round to oval and stain light blue with Wright's stain. The nuclear chromatin is composed of deoxyribonucleic acid *(DNA)* and stains light purple; however, the chromatin becomes more blue with maturity. The cytoplasm of immature cells contains large amounts of ribonucleic acid *(RNA)* and stains blue; with maturity the cytoplasm stains more red. The cytoplasm of young cells is composed of a complex tubular assembly which is concentrated into a relatively light zone adjacent to the nucleus. This assemblage is composed of the Golgi apparatus and is mainly concerned with the synthesis of carbohydrates and packaging of secretions. This perinuclear clear zone is best observed in plasma cells but is present in many immature cells.

Definite granules become evident at the progranulocyte stage. These granules first appear as small, uniform granules and are pink in color. At the myelocyte stage the granules differentiate and become recognizable as neutrophilic, eosinophilic or basophilic granules. As the cell matures the granules tend to become smaller in size.

The cells used for illustrating the maturation sequence are from the bone marrow of normal cats.

I. NORMAL BONE MARROW AND BLOOD CYTOLOGY

Figure 1

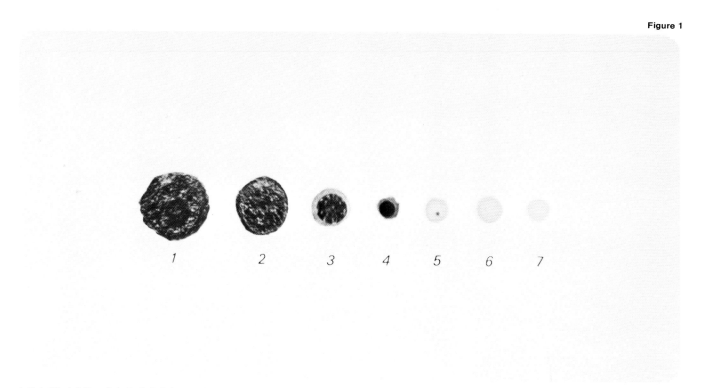

1. Rubriblast 2. Prorubricyte 3. Rubricyte 4. Metarubricyte 5. Basophilic erythrocyte with Howell—Jolly body 6. Basophilic erythrocyte 7. Mature erythrocyte
X 1200

Figure 2

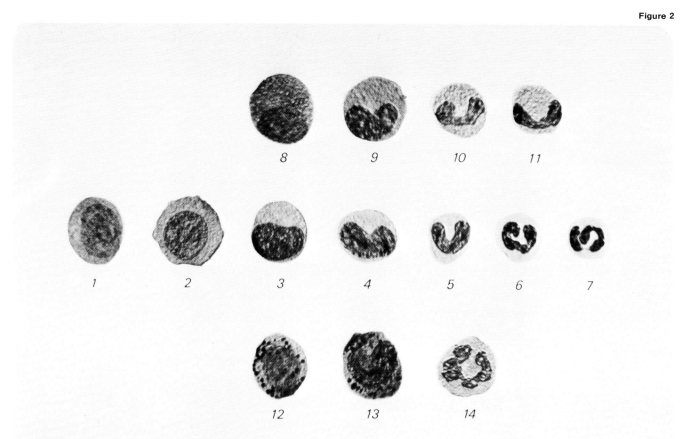

1. Myeloblast with nucleolus 2. Progranulocyte—reddish cytoplasmic granules are scarcely visable, a hint of a retained nucleolus 3. Neutrophilic myelocyte
4. Neutrophilic metamyelocyte 5. Neutrophilic band 6. Monolobed neutrophil 7. Segmented neutrophil 8. Eosinophilic myelocyte 9. Eosinophilic metamyelocyte 10. Eosinophilic band 11. Eosinophil—frequently takes the monolobed form 12. Basophilic myelocyte 13. Basophilic metamyelocyte 14. Basophil—
nucleus, often monolobed granules, small and few in number X 1200

Bone Marrow Cytology

Development of the Erythrocyte

Erythrocytes develop in the bone marrow from the undifferentiated stem cell. Erythrocyte precursor cells can be readily differentiated from the leukocytic precursors by their distinctly round nucleus and the intense basophilia of the cytoplasm. Figure 1 illustrates the normal development of the erythrocyte.

RUBRIBLAST

A large almost perfectly round cell which contains a large round nucleus with a thin rim of royal blue stippled cytoplasm. Light blue nucleoli are present and may be prominent. The nuclear chromatin is rather delicate but stippled. A distinct perinuclear clear area is often observed. Rubriblasts may be differentiated in normal bone marrow.

PRORUBRICYTE

Similar to the rubriblast except smaller in size and nucleoli are absent. The nucleus is round and the chromatin is slightly more coarse in character than the rubriblast. The cytoplasm is predominantly royal blue in color. A perinuclear clear zone is common.

RUBRICYTE

This cell is smaller than the prorubricyte. The nuclear chromatin takes an alternate dark and light streaked pattern, the so-called spoke wheel arrange-ment. The nucleus is round and stains dark purple with blue-black chromatin clumps. The cytoplasm stains intently blue in the early rubricyte but this blue color is gradually diluted out by the pink color of hemoglobin as it matures towards the next stage. This cell can be further subdivided, according to the amount of hemoglobin in the cytoplasm, into basophilic, polychromatic, or normochromatic rubricyte.

METARUBRICYTE

The nucleus has undergone pyknotic degeneration and appears as a dark blue homogeneous mass without any distinct chromatin structure. Hemoglobin is contained within the cytoplasm and imparts considerable pink staining characteristics to the overall basophilic color.

BASOPHILIC ERYTHROCYTE

This is an anucleate erythrocyte that has slight basophilia of the cytoplasm. They are larger than the mature erythrocytes. When stained with a supravital stain such as new methylene blue* some basophilic erythrocytes show evidence of a network of blue fibers. This network is precipitated RNA and any cell so stained with a supravital stain is called a reticulocyte (Fig. 12-10).

ERYTHROCYTE

The mature cells of the peripheral blood that stain pink in color.

Development of the Granulocytes
(Neutrophils, Eosinophils and Basophils)

Granulocytes develop in the bone marrow from the undifferentiated stem cell. Granulocytes are readily differentiated from the nucleated erythrocytes by their fine, reticulated chromatin structure and bluish pink, readily folded cytoplasm. Figure 2 illustrates the development of the granulocytes.

The morphologic descriptions described below are general characteristics that apply to the cat. Species variations and the more mature granulocytes are illustrated with photographs in the section on "Description of Leukocytes in Peripheral Blood."

MYELOBLAST

These are large cells which have a round or oval purple staining nucleus with delicate, reticulated chromatin strands. Generally one to occasionally two pale blue nucleoli are evident. The cytoplasm

*New Methylene Blue—(Basic Blue 24), Matheson, Coleman and Bell; East Rutherford, New Jersey 07073.

Development of the Granulocytes *con't.*

stains bluish pink and contains no specific granules. It may be difficult to distinguish myeloblasts from other "blast cells."

PROGRANULOCYTE

This cell has distinct small pinkish granules in the cytoplasm. The nuclear chromatin is delicate and similar to the myeloblast, only more coarse and occasionally contains nucleoli. The cytoplasm generally stains less intently blue than the myeloblast. The characteristic cytoplasmic pinkish granules identify the progranulocyte.

MYELOCYTE

A progranulocyte becomes a myelocyte when the granules have differentiated and are recognized as neutrophilic, eosinophilic or basophilic granules. The nucleus is round and frequently eccentrically placed; nucleoli are absent. A perinuclear clear zone (Golgi apparatus) may be present and the cytoplasm stains gray-blue and may contain a few vacuoles. The myelocytes and all subsequent granulocytes should be distinguished as neutrophilic, eosinophilic or basophilic according to the color of their specific granules. Neutrophilic granules are barely discernible and are to be contrasted with the more definite eosinophilic and basophilic granules. The eosinophilic myelocyte contains numerous acidophilic rod-shaped granules and a few very small basophilic granules (Fig. 2). The morphology of the immature cat basophils uniquly contain small round pink granules and a few larger round black granules.

METAMYELOCYTE

This cell is distinguished from the myelocyte by its indented kidney-shaped nucleus. The nuclear chromatin becomes more coarse. The cytoplasm stains less intently blue than the myelocyte. Cytoplasmic neutrophilic, eosinophilic or basophilic granules are present.

BAND

When the nucleus becomes horseshoe-shaped, it is designated a band cell. The nucleus has smooth, parallel sides with only a slight indentation. The diameter of the midportion of the nucleus may be equal to or often less than the ends making the band appear as a coiled dumbell. The chromatin stains purplish blue and is coarse. A band cell may be neutrophilic, eosinophilic or basophilic depending upon its staining properties. These more mature eosinophils and basophils are described under "Description of Leukocytes in Peripheral Blood" for each particular species.

MONOLOBED NEUTROPHIL

The monolobed neutrophil is the most common granulocyte that occurs in the peripheral blood of domestic animals. The nucleus is intermediate in shape between the band and segmented neutrophil. The nuclear membrane is rough and ragged but nuclear filaments are absent. The nuclear chromatin is coarse. The cytoplasm is light pink and may or may not contain fine pinkish staining neutrophilic granules.

SEGMENTED NEUTROPHIL

A cell containing specific neutrophilic granules where the lobes of the nucleus are connected by fine nuclear filaments.

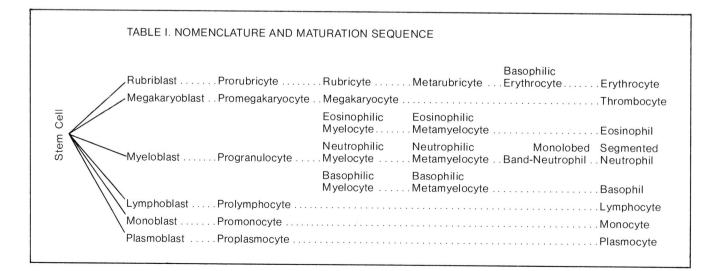

TABLE I. NOMENCLATURE AND MATURATION SEQUENCE

Stem Cell						
Rubriblast	Prorubricyte	Rubricyte	Metarubricyte	Basophilic Erythrocyte	Erythrocyte	
Megakaryoblast	Promegakaryocyte	Megakaryocyte			Thrombocyte	
		Eosinophilic Myelocyte	Eosinophilic Metamyelocyte		Eosinophil	
Myeloblast	Progranulocyte	Neutrophilic Myelocyte	Neutrophilic Metamyelocyte	Monolobed Band-Neutrophil	Segmented Neutrophil	
		Basophilic Myelocyte	Basophilic Metamyelocyte		Basophil	
Lymphoblast	Prolymphocyte				Lymphocyte	
Monoblast	Promonocyte				Monocyte	
Plasmoblast	Proplasmocyte				Plasmocyte	

Development of the Thrombocyte and Plasmocyte

MEGAKARYOCYTE

Megakaryocytes are the largest cells in the bone marrow (50-150 microns in diameter) and are very prominent (Figure 3). Promegakaryocytes have non-granular cytoplasm and are to be contrasted with the mature megakaryocytes which contain small purplish red cytoplasmic granules. The nuclei of the mature megakaryocytes are large, twisted, irregularly shaped, often multinucleated and connected by nuclear strands. The cytoplasm is abundant and light blue with indistinct cell borders.

THROMBOCYTES

Thrombocytes or platelets are small round, non-nucleated cells that are considered to be cytoplasmic fragments of megakaryocytes. They contribute to hemostasis by providing coagulation factors (platelet factor 3) as well as forming a hemostatic plug which seals breaks in small blood vessels. They are extremely variable in size and shape. The cytoplasm is pale blue and contains purplish granules. Giant and cigar shaped forms are not uncommon especially in the cat. Thrombocytes tend to adhere to each other, thus clumps of platelets are often found at the feather edge of blood smears.

PLASMOCYTES

Plasma cells constitute less than 1% of the nucleated cells of the bone marrow and are only rarely observed in blood smears. Plasma cells are round to ellipsoidal shaped with an eccentrically placed nucleus (Figure 4). The nucleus contains large clumps of chromatin which resemble the nuclear pattern found in the rubricyte. Nucleoli are absent in all but the rarely observed plasmoblast. The cytoplasm contains abundant RNA and stains royal blue. There is a well defined perinuclear clear zone which consists of concentrically arranged endoplasmic reticulum with the associated Golgi apparatus. Plasmocytes produce immunoglobulins (antibodies).

Figure 3/ Megakaryocytes   Figure 3 / 1

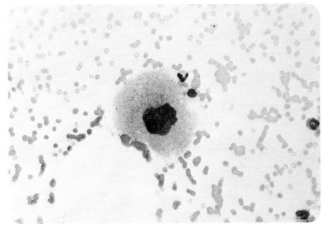

Examples of mature megakaryocytes with small purplish red cytoplasmic granules X 1000

Figure 3 / 2

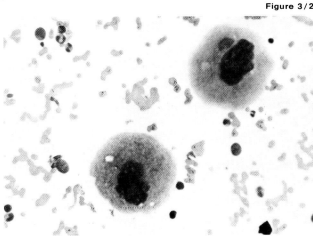

See Figure 3/1

Figure 4/ Plasmocytes   Figure 4 / 1

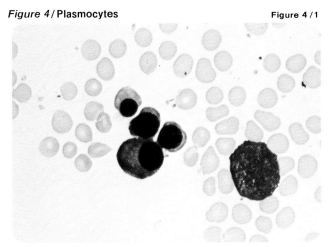

1. Plasma cell with eccentric nucleus that resembles the nuclei of the 3 nucleated erythrocytes above. Smudged free nucleus on right. X 1000.

Figure 4 / 2

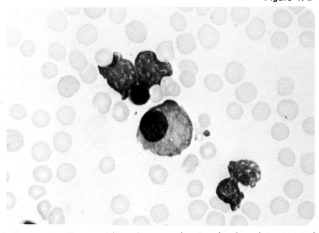

2. Plasmocyte with eccentric nucleus, prominent perinuclear clear zone and royal blue cytoplasm. Surrounded by smudged cells and a metarubricyte. X 1000.

Miscellaneous Bone Marrow Cells
Fixed Tissue Cells

In addition to the cells already described there are various types of cells that are uncommonly observed in marrow aspirates. These cells are immobile and hence called fixed tissue cells (Figure 5). Fixed tissue cells are larger than the other marrow cells, except the megakaryocyte, and often have indistinct cytoplasmic margins. The nuclei of these cells are round and only rarely fold. The chromatin is coarse, linear and appears "spaghetti-like." One or two distinct pale blue nucleoli are apparent. The cytoplasm is pale blue and contains various numbers of pinkish granules.

RETICULUM CELLS
These are large cells with abundant pale blue cytoplasm. The cytoplasm may contain a few pinkish granules. The nuclear chromatin is linear and "spaghetti-like" with 1 to 2 light blue nucleoli. Reticulum cells are quite fragile and few remain intact in normal marrow aspirates. Free reticulum cell nuclei with their prominent nucleoli are common in normal marrow.

TISSUE NEUTROPHIL
Morphology similar to reticulum cell except that granules are more numerous, larger and acidophilic.

PHAGOCYTIC HISTIOCYTE
A large cell with indistinct cytoplasmic borders. Cytoplasmic vacuoles are prominent. The nucleus is similar in appearance to the reticulum cell but smaller. This cell is identifiable because of the phagocytized particles within its cytoplasm. Erythrocytes and nuclear fragments are commonly observable phagocytized materials.

OSTEOBLASTS AND OSTEOCLASTS
Osteoblasts are similar in appearance to plasmocytes but are much larger. Osteoblasts have ample cytoplasm with an eccentrically placed nucleus. The nuclei contain 1 or 2 nucleoli and the chromatin pattern is coarse and linear. The basophilic cytoplasm is abundant and frequently, like the plasma cell, contains a perinuclear clear zone.

Osteoclasts are giant multinucleated cells seen infrequently in the bone marrow of adult animals. The number of nuclei is quite variable. The nuclei are round and do not touch one another. This is to be contrasted with the nuclei of megakaryocytes which are connected by nuclear strands. One nucleolus is generally found in each osteoclast nucleus. The chromatin is dense. The cytoplasm is abundant, indistinct and granular with numerous pinkish granules of various sizes.

Figure 5/ Fixed Tissue Cells   Figure 5/1

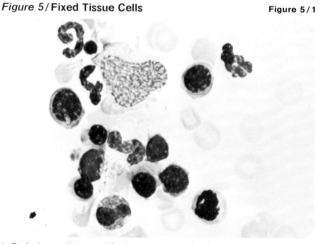

1. Reticulum cell, located in the upper left, with linear chromatin and 1 nucleolus; surrounded by nucleated erythrocytes and granulocytes. X 1000

Figure 5 / Fixed Tissue Cells

Figure 5 / 2

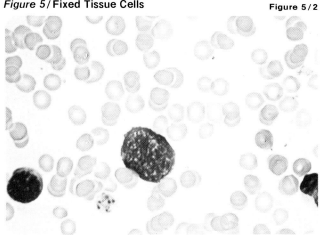

2. Free nucleus of reticulum cell. X 1000

Figure 5 / 5

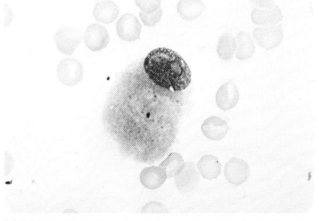

5. A large osteoblast with ample cytoplasm and eccentrically placed nucleus. X 1000

Figure 5 / 3

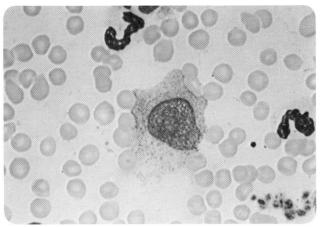

3. Tissue neutrophil with definite nucleolus and acidophilic cytoplasmic granules. X 1000

Figure 5 / 6

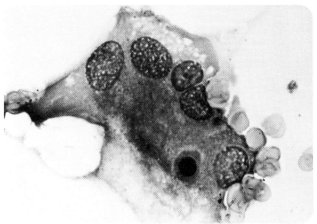

6. Osteoclast with 5 separated nuclei; rubricyte in background. X 1000

Figure 5 / 4

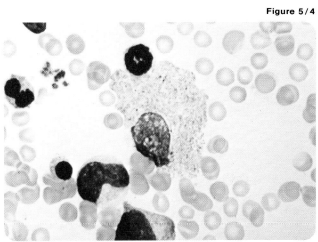

4. Tissue eosinophil with refractile rod-shaped cytoplasmic granules X 1000

Figure 5 / 7

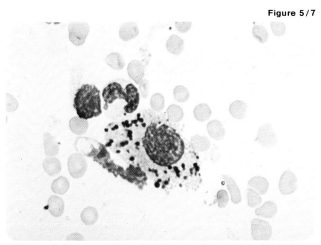

7. Phagocytic histiocyte with nuclear fragments in cytoplasm. X 1000

Description of Erythrocytes in Peripheral Blood

Canine

At birth, the dog's erythrocyte is approximately 10 microns in diameter; these large red blood cells are gradually replaced until about 6 months of age when the erythrocytes approximate the normal adult value of 7.0 microns. Having the largest diameter, the dog's RBC can normally exhibit slight variations in shape. This cell normally is in the shape of a biconcave disk and when examined on the blood smear has a well-defined area of central pallor (Fig. 23-2). Rouleaux (RBC's adhering to each other in the form of a roll or column) are commonly present. An occasional folded cell or target cell (Fig. 23-2), basophilic erythrocyte, or metarubricyte may be encountered in a normal canine blood smear. Crenated erythrocytes, irregular margins appearing as sharp points, are observed in improperly dried blood slides and in blood slides made from anticoagulant blood. For good blood morphology, fresh blood slides without anticoagulant must be prepared.

Feline

The red cell is large at birth gradually becoming smaller until it reaches its mean adult diameter of 6 microns. The small size of the erythrocyte precludes development of central pallor. Slight anisocytosis, rouleau formation and crenation are rather characteristic of feline erythrocytes. A few Howell-Jolly bodies (Fig. 2) and nucleated red blood cells may be observed in the peripheral blood in the normal or stressed cat. Erythrocyte refractile bodies or ER bodies (also called Heinz bodies) are commonly noticed in cat erythrocytes. With Wright's Stain, these appear as small, circular pale areas in erythrocytes (Fig. 13-14) and are thought to be altered hemoglobin. With new methylene blue these bodies stain blue-black (Fig. 13-15). As many as 10% of erythrocytes may be affected in normal healthy cats.

Equine

In the adult horse as a comparison, the mean erythrocyte diameter is approximately 5 microns. Anisocytosis is only slight. Rouleau formation is most marked in the horse, only taking a few minutes for the erythrocytes to separate completely from the plasma. A few Howell-Jolly bodies may be found in erythrocytes.

Description of Leukocytes in Peripheral Blood

Canine

NEUTROPHIL

Monolobed neutrophils are the most common cells in the peripheral blood of the dog. The nucleus is irregular and ragged with true filaments being rare. The chromatin is coarse and clumped while the cytoplasm often stains pale pink with slight diffuse granulation.

NEUTROPHILIC BANDS AND METAMYELOCYTES

Bands are only rarely found in the peripheral blood of normal dogs and then comprise less than 2% of the leukocytes. The nucleus is horseshoe in shape and the ends are often round and larger than the midportion of the nucleus. Metamyelocytes are not found in normal canine blood smears.

LYMPHOCYTES

This is the second most common cell found in peripheral blood of the dog. It is imperative that the normal morphology of these cells is known since anything that differs from normal is often called atypical and may suggest a diagnosis of lymphosarcoma. (See PATHOLOGIC CYTOLOGY — Lymphosarcoma.)

Small lymphocyte. The small lymphocyte has a nuclear diameter that is equal to or slightly greater than that of the canine erythrocyte (7 to 10 microns in diameter). The nucleus is round to slightly indented with heavy coarse clumps of chromatin. With Wright's stain the chromatin stains dark purple; no nucleolus is present. The sky blue cytoplasm is scanty and frequently indiscernible.

Large lymphocyte. Large lymphocytes vary greatly in size. Both the nucleus and cytoplasm are more abundant than the small lymphocyte. The nucleus is round to slightly indented or kidney-shaped. The chromatin is more reticular and stains less intense. Chromatin clumps are present while nucleoli are absent. The nucleus is eccentrically placed in abundant pale blue cytoplasm. A few well-defined large pinkish cytoplasmic granules (lysosomes) may be observed.

Figure 6/ Normal Dog Leukocytes   Figure 6/1

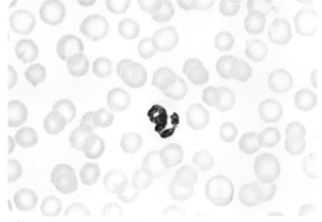

1. Monolobed neutrophil X 1000

Figure 6/2

2. Neutrophilic band X 1000

Figure 6/3

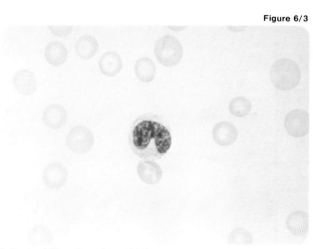

3. Neutrophilic metamyelocyte X 1000

13

Description of Leukocytes in Peripheral Blood *con't.*

Lymphocytes are fragile, easily molded cells. The cytoplasmic margins are often indented by erythrocytes. Mechanical injury may cause the cytoplasmic membranes to appear stellate or spindle shaped. Because of this folding, the cytoplasmic margins may stain more intensely blue than the cytoplasm.

Immunocyte. Lymphocytes transform into immunocytes in the presence of antigen. Immunocytes are recognized by their mature lymphocyte-like nucleus and intense cytoplasmic basophilia. Immunocytes synthesize immune globulins and their presence in peripheral blood indicates an immune response.

MONOCYTE
Monocytes are the largest cells in peripheral blood. The nuclear shape is variable but is generally lobulated. A large kidney-shaped nucleus is rather characteristic but superimposed nuclear lobes are not uncommon. The nucleus may resemble a band neutrophil or metamyelocyte and in this case other morphologic characteristics are required for identification. Nuclear chromatin in the monocyte is diffuse and more loose than the clumped chromatin of a lymphocyte. Nucleoli are not evident. The monocyte can frequently be identified by its characteristic blue-gray cytoplasm. Cytoplasmic vacuoles are often present and vary in size giving it a frothy appearance. Monocytes are motile cells and reveal blunt cytoplasmic pseudopods which are agranular and stain a faint blue color. Numerous fine, lightly stained pinkish granules are diffusely scattered throughout the cytoplasm. The cytoplasmic appearance is often referred to as having a "ground glass" appearance. Monocytes which have phagocytized erythrocytes or nuclear debris may occasionally be noted at the feather edge of the blood slide.

BASOPHIL
The basophil of the dog is rarely recognized because of its unusual morphologic features. The nucleus is often sausage-shaped to highly segmented and is readily discernible. The granules are few in number and stain purplish to blue-black. The cytoplasm is gray-blue and often contains small vacuoles. Degranulated basophils may be observed and are often confused with monocytes.

THROMBOCYTES
These cells exhibit variation in size, shape and color. The thrombocyte is generally a small, pale blue cell which contains a few purplish granules. Occasionally, they reach giant proportions with abundant, irregular cytoplasmic margins. Thrombocytes that are huge in size or clumped often interfere with and cause the leukocyte count to read high if an electronic cell counter* is used.

EOSINOPHIL
The shape and degree of granulation in the canine eosinophil is extremely variable. The granules may be uniform in size or may vary considerably with small and large granules present in the same cell. With intense stimulation these granules seem to coalesce until 1 or 2 huge granules are evident. These eosinophilic granules stain less intently in the dog and have approximately the same staining characteristics as the mature erythrocyte. There may be small vacuoles in some canine eosinophils. The nuclear structure is similar to the neutrophil but may be partially obscured by the eosinophilic granules.

*Coulter Counter, Coulter Electronics, Inc. Hialeah, Florida.

Figure 6/ Normal Dog Leukocytes

Figure 6/4

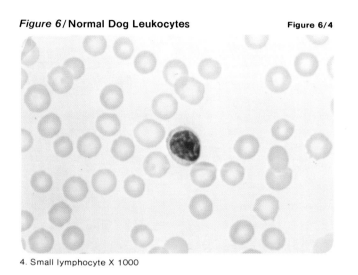

4. Small lymphocyte X 1000

Figure 6/5

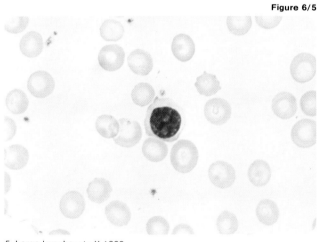

5. Large lymphocyte X 1000

Figure 6/6

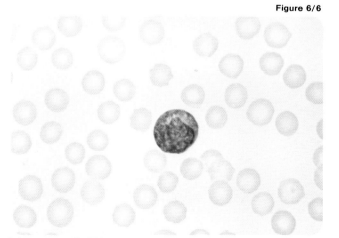

6. Immunocyte X 1000

Figure 6/7

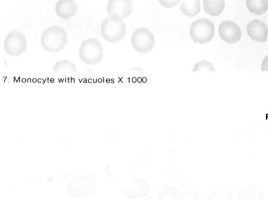

7. Monocyte with vacuoles X 1000

Figure 6/8

8. Eosinophil with granules of varying sizes, nucleus often unsegmented X 1000

Figure 6/9

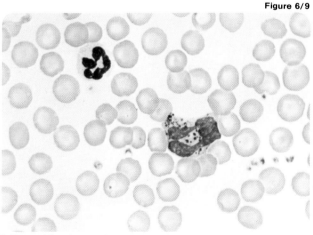

9. Neutrophil and basophil; note small anuclear thrombocytes in lower right X 1000

Description of Leukocytes in Peripheral Blood *con't.*

Feline

NEUTROPHIL
The nuclear structure is similar to the dog neutrophil (Figure 7). The cytoplasm is often a blue-gray without prominent neutrophilic granules. Small basophilic granules may appear in the cytoplasm often at the edge of the neutrophils. A few of these granules, so called Dohle bodies, can be observed in normal cat's neutrophils and are thought to be altered RNA. This is considered to be a sign of "mild toxicity" in the cat. More severe signs of "toxicity" include basophilia of cytoplasm and increased size of neutrophils with foamy cytoplasm (Fig. 14-2).

EOSINOPHIL
In the cat, eosinophilic granules are rod-like and numerous, often partially obscuring the nucleus.

BASOPHIL
The cat basophil is often classified as an eosinophil. The size of this cell and the numbers of granules are similar; however, the granules of the basophil are smaller and stain a definite lavender color. The cytoplasm likewise appears lavender. Degranulated basophils are common. The nucleus may be sausage-shaped to highly segmented.

THROMBOCYTES
The cat's thrombocytes are very pleomorphic. Giant forms as large as small lymphocytes are commonly seen. They may be very elongated or appear cigar-shaped.

OTHER CELLS
Lymphocytes and monocytes have the same general characteristics as described for the dog.

Figure 7 / Normal Cat Leukocytes Figure 7/1

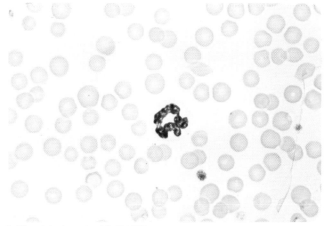

1. Monolobed neutrophil. X 1000

Figure 7/2

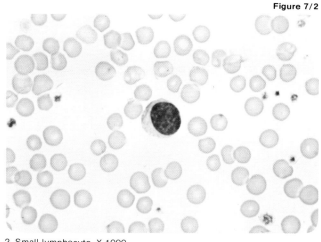

2. Small lymphocyte. X 1000

Figure 7/3

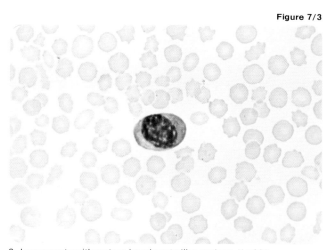

3. Immunocyte with mature lymphocyte-like nucleus. X 1000

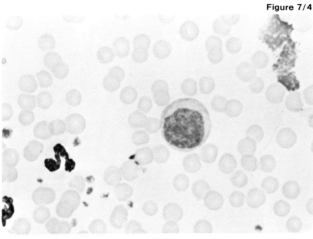

4. Immunocyte with large nucleus. X 1000

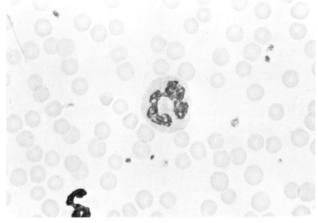

7. Basophil with subtle lavender granules. X 1000

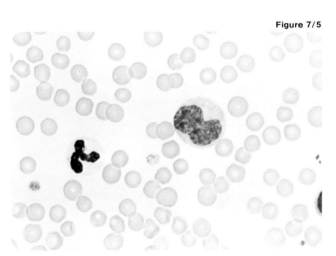

5. Neutrophil and monocyte. X 1000

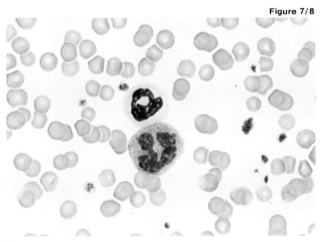

8. Basophil and monolobed neutrophil. X 1000

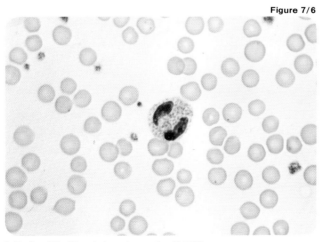

6. Eosinophil with rod-shaped granules. X 1000

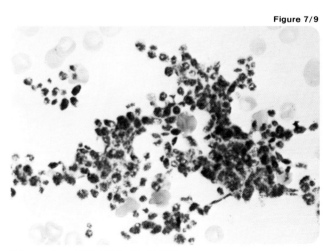

9. Large clump of thrombocytes. X 1000

Comparative Leukocyte Morphology of the Horse

Equine

NEUTROPHIL
The nuclear chromatin is coarse and heavily clumped (Figure 8). The cytoplasm is filled with fine, pinkish dust-like neutrophilic granules. Band neutrophils are only rarely observed in the peripheral blood of the horse.

LYMPHOCYTE
Most are of the small lymphocyte type but some are large with abundant, pale blue cytoplasm. The latter cells have a smooth rather homogeneous nucleus. A few small azurophilic granules may be present.

MONOCYTE
A large cell with a kidney-shaped nucleus. Resembles the dog's monocyte.

EOSINOPHIL
The horse has the most distinctive eosinophilic granules. They are very large, generally round to oblong in shape and stain an intense orange-red color. They completely pack the cytoplasm, may partially obscure the nucleus and alter the cytoplasmic membrane such that the membrane conforms to the shape of the granules. The nucleus is generally homogeneous in appearance taking a band-like shape.

BASOPHIL
The granules are irregular in size and shape; some being oval and others rod-shaped. The majority of these granules stain dark purple but others stain lighter purple. The granules may be irregularly scattered or completely pack the cytoplasm causing the nucleus to be partially obscured. The nucleus is large, homogeneous without abundant nuclear chromatin clumping, and often takes the band shape.

THROMBOCYTES
They are rather indistinct in the horse with irregular barely discernible cytoplasmic membranes. The granules are indistinct and few in number.

Figure 8 / **Normal Horse Leukocytes**

Figure 8/1

1. Neutrophil and small lymphocyte. X 1000

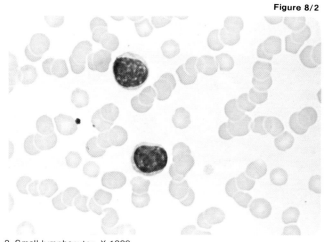

Figure 8/2

2. Small lymphocytes. X 1000

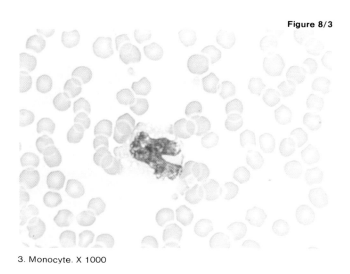

Figure 8/3

3. Monocyte. X 1000

Problem Cells—Differential Features

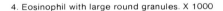

Figure 8/4

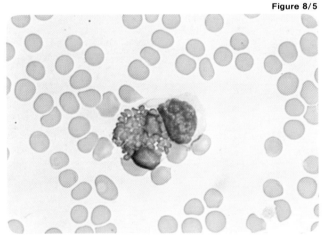

4. Eosinophil with large round granules. X 1000

Figure 8/5

5. Eosinophil and large lymphocyte. X 1000

Figure 8/6

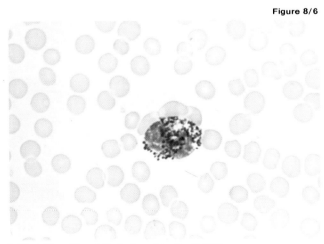

6. Basophil and few delicate thrombocytes. X 1000

Several principles are helpful when trying to identify problem cells in peripheral blood. First, find "classic" examples of granulocytes, lymphocytes and monocytes in peripheral blood. Study these cells carefully paying particular attention to staining characteristics of both nucleus and cytoplasm as well as structure of the nuclear chromatin. After identifying the morphologic characteristics of the various cells on the particular slide, observe the problem cells. Comparing the morphologic features of the problem cells with other positively identified cells will permit accurate classification. In general, there are fewer immature cells than mature cells in peripheral blood. Thus, it is expected, with the exception of leukemia, to identify more mature cells in the peripheral blood. For example, many monolobed kidney-shaped cells are found in the peripheral blood. The question is whether they are metamyelocytes or monocytes. If they are metamyelocytes, one should find increased numbers of bands, unless granulocytic leukemia exists. The absence of bands helps to identify these cells as monocytes. Cells may be and often must be identified according to "the company they keep."

Monocyte vs. Large Lymphocyte

Monocytes are the most difficult to identify and differentiate from other peripheral blood cells. They can be confused with large lymphocytes (Figure 9). The features that are the most helpful in identification of a monocyte are the vacuolated, dull blue-gray abundant cytoplasm and the kidney-shaped nucleus with its fine to reticulated nuclear chromatin. The large nucleus of the lymphocyte is generally round to slightly indented. The nuclear chromatin is clumped rather than reticulated. The cytoplasm is sky-blue not blue-gray and only rarely does it contain vacuoles. Occasionally a lymphocyte will contain rather large, randomly distributed, azurophilic cytoplasmic granules. These are readily distinguished from the uniform and small granules of the monocyte.

Problem Cells—Differential Features *con't.*

Monocyte vs. Metamyelocyte

A classic monocyte, as described above, must be first recognized on the particular blood slide and then compared with known neutrophilic bands and metamyelocytes in the same or adjacent fields (Figure 10). The cytoplasm of the metamyelocyte is generally lighter and more reddish staining when compared to the bluish, often vacuolated cytoplasm of the monocyte. The nucleus of the monocyte is often multilobulated; this is not seen with metamyelocytes. Pseudopods may be found with monocytes but not metamyelocytes. If bands are absent, the monolobed kidney-shaped cell in question is likely to be a monocyte.

Small Lymphocyte vs. Rubricyte

The nucleus of the small lymphocyte is usually round to slightly indented and eccentrically placed (Figure 11). The nuclear chromatin is splotchy and clumped, while the cytoplasm is light blue and sparse. Rubricytes are generally round cells with a distinct rim of cytoplasm. The nuclear chromatin is coarse and takes an alternate dark and light streaked pattern. With Wright's Stain the nucleus of the lymphocyte stains predominately a purple color; the rubricyte nucleus stains more blue to black in color. Individual cells may have to be classified by association with predominant cells.

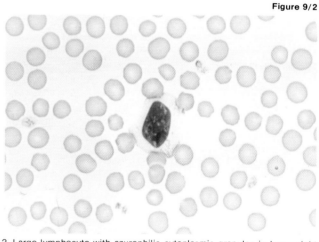

Figure 9/ Monocytes vs. Large Lymphocyte   Figure 9/1

1. Two monocytes with kidney-shaped nuclei, vacuoles and blue-gray cytoplasm. X 1000

Figure 9/2

2. Large lymphocyte with azurophilic cytoplasmic granules in lower right. X 1000

Figure 9/3

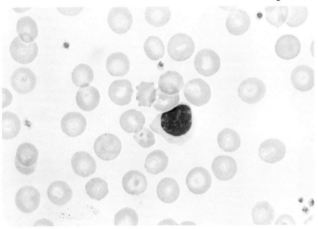

3. Lymphocyte with slightly compressed nucleus and cytoplasm. X 1000

Figure 10/3

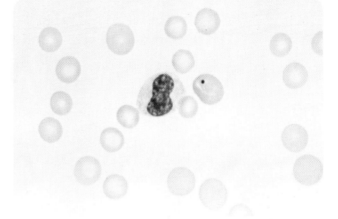

3. Metamyelocyte next to Howell-Jolly body. X 1000

Figure 10/1

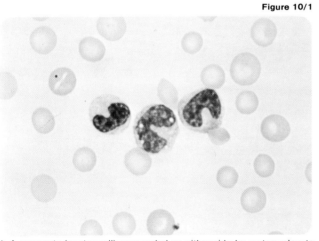

1. A monocyte (center cell) surrounded on either side by metamyelocyte. Cytoplasm of metamyelocyte is more red than of a monocyte. X 1000

Figure 11/1

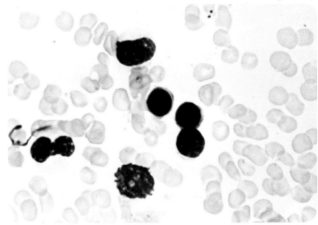

1. Bone marrow comparing small lymphocyte (lower) with 2 metarubricytes immediately above lymphocyte. The uppermost cell is a lymphocyte, followed counter clockwise by a band neutrophil and free reticulum cell nucleus. X 1000

Figure 10/2

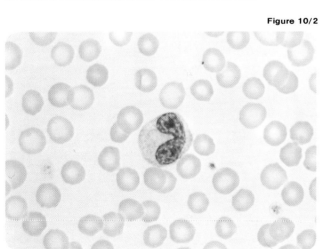

2. Monocyte with blue-grey cytoplasm but without vacuoles. X 1000

Figure 11/2

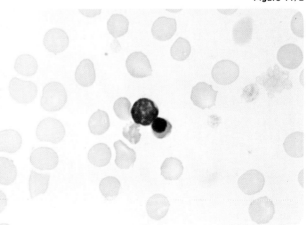

2. A metarubricyte (lower right) is touching a small lymphocyte. X 1000

II. Pathologic Cytology

This section emphasizes the use of the blood and bone marrow slide in making a diagnosis or suggesting alternate diagnoses. One can identify abnormalities in the red blood cells, leukocytes and thrombocytes by examination of the peripheral blood slide.

A brief description regarding the classification of anemia, causes of leukocytosis, leukopenia, thrombocytopenia and classification of myeloproliferative disease is given. This is over-simplified, yet when this information is correlated with blood and bone marrow morphology, it will suggest certain diagnoses. For example, Figure 27 shows small, pale stained canine erythrocytes. This indicates iron deficiency anemia and is caused by chronic blood loss. Specific causes of chronic blood loss include bloody diarrhea, gastrointestinal ulcers, bleeding neoplasms and blood-sucking parasites. This information is definitely helpful, and when correlated with the history and physical findings of a specific case, may suggest a definitive diagnosis as well as a specific treatment.

ERYTHROCYTE ABNORMALITIES

Classification of Anemia

There are many different methods for classifying anemias. In this monograph a simple etiologic classification will be used. Anemias are divided into two broad groups based on bone marrow response to the anemia. The first group will be called regenerative anemia; in this case there is evidence of increased red blood cell production in the peripheral blood and bone marrow. This category can be subdivided into blood loss and blood destruction (hemolysis) anemias. The second broad group will be called non-regenerative anemia. Here the increase in red cell precursors in blood and bone marrow is less than expected for the degree of anemia. Subgroups of this category would include anemia of infection, anemia of chronic renal disease, nutritional anemias (iron, B_{12}, folic acid), anemias caused by certain drugs and anemias associated with lymphosarcoma and myeloproliferative disease.

Anoxia is the general stimulus for red cell production. In the simplest sense, anoxia causes the kidney to release a hormone, erythropoietin, that stimulates the bone marrow to increase red cell production. Signs of regeneration are manifested in the peripheral blood of the dog and cat 3-4 days following stimulation. Signs noted on the blood slide include:

Reticulocytosis—blue reticulum in supravitally stained erythrocytes (new methylene blue).

Polychromasia—large, blue anucleated erythrocytes.

Anisocytosis—variation in size of erythrocytes.

Nucleated erythrocytes (NRBC's)—nucleus retained within erythrocyte.

Howell-Jolly Bodies—small, round erythrocytic nuclear fragments.

Polychromasia and reticulocytosis in the dog and cat are the best indicators of regenerative anemia. The dog is considered to be the best responder. The cat responds, as evidenced by polychromasia and reticulocytosis, to a lesser degree. Regenerative signs in peripheral blood (polychromasia or reticulocytosis) are not observed in the horse. Hence, with the cat and horse, signs of increased red cell production may be lacking, especially if the anemia is not severe. In this case, evaluation of anemia must be accomplished by evaluation of the bone marrow for increased erythrogenesis.

If peripheral blood reticulocytes or bone marrow erythroid cells are less than expected for the degree of anemia and if the history indicates that the animal has been ill for more than 4 days, the anemia is classified as non-regenerative.

The degree by which the dog responds (polychromasia and reticulocytosis) may offer a clue as to the specific cause for the anemia. Blood loss externally, for example, results in a minimal response (Fig. 23) while blood loss into a body cavity or by hemolysis causes marked regenerative response (Fig. 28-30).

Figure 12 / Pathologic Erythrocytes

Figure 12/1

1. Crenated erythrocytes, margins appearing as sharp points. May result when blood slides dry slowly or as a normal process in aging of red cells. X 1000

Figure 12/2

2. Acanthocytes, erythrocytes with blunt projections, thought to be a membrane defect; commonly noted in kidney disease, splenic disease (hemangiosarcoma) autoimmune hemolytic anemia and occasionally in liver disease. X 1000

Figure 12/3

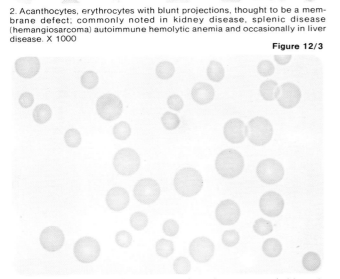

3. Anisocytosis, variation in erythrocyte size; when accompanied by polychromasia erythrogenesis is indicated. X 1000

Figure 12/4

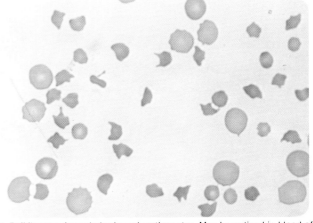

4. Basophilic stippling, blue staining granules in central erythrocyte and poikilocytes. In the dog, the presence of basophilic stippled erythrocytes and nucleated erythrocytes, in the absence of severe anemia, suggest a diagnosis of lead toxicosis. X 1000

Figure 12/5

5. Poikilocytes, irregularly shaped erythrocytes. May be noticed in blood of anemic animals and indicate either improper production or premature destruction of erythrocytes. Poikilocytosis may be noted in renal disease, splenic disease and blood loss anemias. X 1000

Figure 12/6

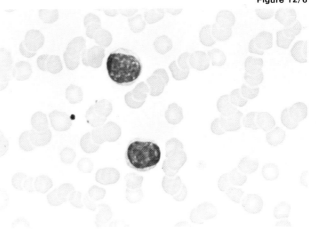

6. Rouleau (plural, rouleaux), erythrocytes in a roll or column. Rouleau is most pronounced in horse blood. X 1000

Pathologic Erythrocytes

Figure 12/Pathologic Erythrocytes

Figure 12/7

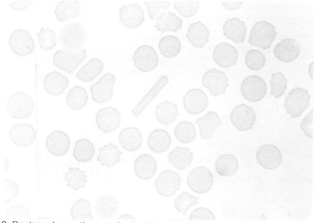

7. Spherocytes, dense spherical canine erythrocytes lacking normal biconcave shape. Polychromasia, large blue erythrocytes. Spherocytes indicate red cell membrane abnormality associated with an increased permeability to sodium ions, and is associated with autoimmune mechanism hemolysis. Polychromasia indicates evidence of erythrogenesis. X 1000

Figure 12/8

8. Rectangular erythrocyte in dog blood, rarely noted and significance unknown. X 1000

Figure 12/9

9. Target cells, irregularly shaped erythrocytes with the appearance of a target. Target cells are observed along with polychromasia in regenerative anemias. However, their appearance without polychromasia, suggests the possibility of kidney, liver or splenic disease. X 1000

Figure 12/10

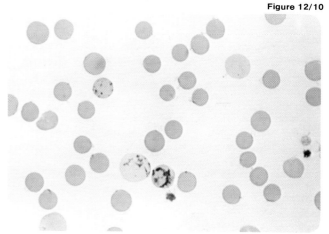

10. Reticulocytes, blue reticulum stained with new methylene blue and counterstained with Wright's stain. Reticulocytes are the best indicator of regenerative anemia in peripheral blood. X 1000

Figure 12/11

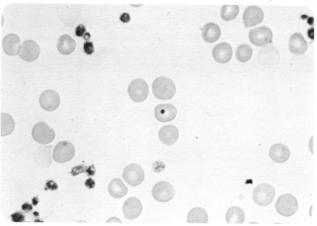

11. Howell-Jolly body, a nuclear fragment. May be noted in regenerative anemias; however, if numerous suggest hyposplenism. X 1000

Figure 12/12

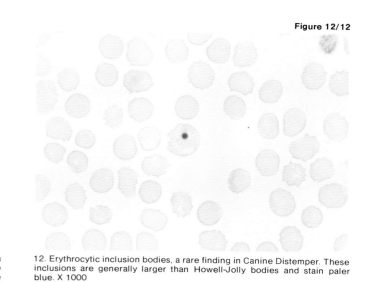

12. Erythrocytic inclusion bodies, a rare finding in Canine Distemper. These inclusions are generally larger than Howell-Jolly bodies and stain paler blue. X 1000

Figure 12 / Pathologic Erythrocytes

Figure 12/13

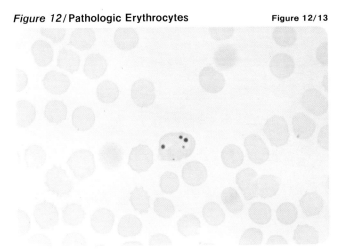

13. Same as 12, except numerous inclusions in one erythrocyte. X 1000

Figure 12/14

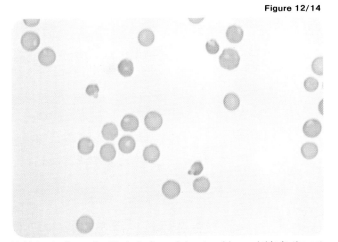

14. Heinz bodies, refractile inclusions of denatured hemoglobin in the cat. These inclusions often protrude causing bulging of erythrocyte. The oxidant drug, methylene blue, produced these changes in the cat's erythrocytes. X 1000

Figure 12/15

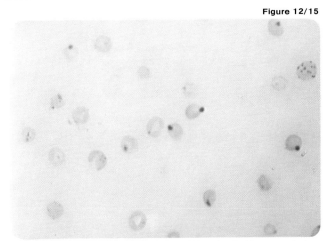

15. Heinz bodies in cat, same as 14 except slide stained with new methylene blue. X 1000

Figure 12/16

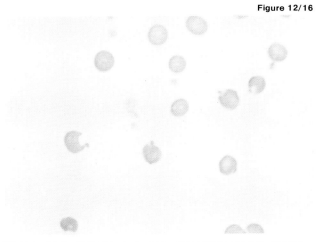

16. Heinz bodies in the horse caused by phenothiazine toxicity. X 1000

Figure 12/17

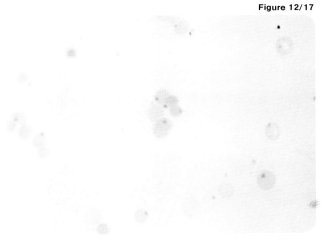

17. Same as 16 except slide stained with new methylene blue. X 1000

Figure 12/18

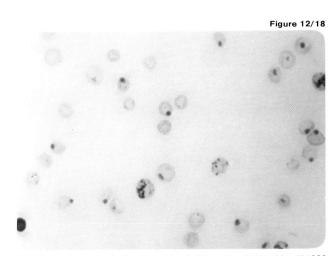

18. Heinz bodies and reticulocytes, stained with new methylene blue. X 1000

25

Blood Parasites

Figure 13/1

Figure 13/2

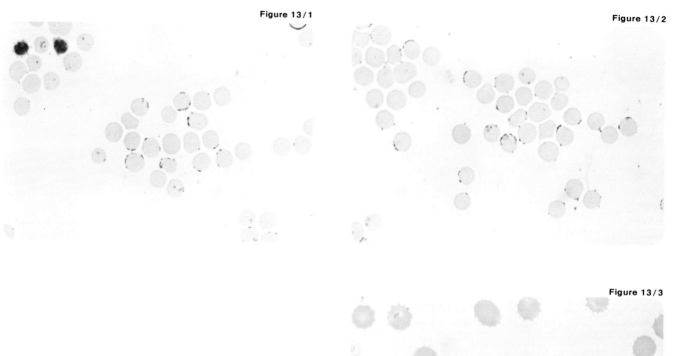

Figure 13/3

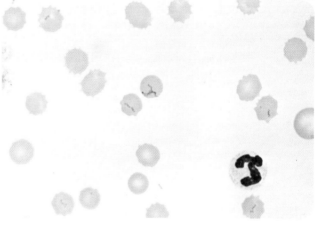

Figure 13/4

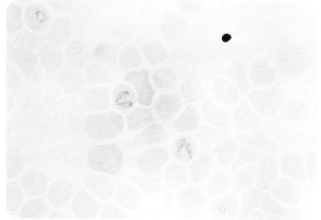

Figure 13 / 5

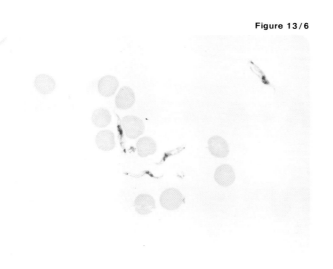

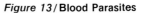

Figure 13 / Blood Parasites

1. *Haemobartonella felis*, cocci or rods at the margin of erythrocytes. A few ring forms can be observed in upper left. X 1000

2. *Haemobartonella felis*, organisms at margin of erythrocytes and a few scattered over erythrocyte surface. Haemobartonella organisms are most often noted in secondary disease conditions. Chronic infections and leukemias cause debility which provides ideal conditions for the entrance of haemobartonella organisms. X 1000

3. *Haemobartonella canis*, long chains on the surface of erythrocytes. This organism may become apparent when the spleen is diseased (lymphosarcoma), or following splenectomy. X 1000

4. *Babesia canis*, pairs of tear drop shaped parasites. An erythrocyte in upper left contains one trophozoite. X 1000

5. *Babesia caballi*, numerous tear drop shaped organisms in erythrocytes of a horse. Occasionally polyangular forms and odd shaped developmental stages with long filaments may appear in erythrocytes. X 1000

6. *Trypanosoma congolense*, from horse of Kenya, East Africa. Mammalian trypanosomes take the shape of an elongated flattened blade. The small rounded kinetoplast is in close proximity to the flagellum. The nucleus is often located near the center. X 1000

7. *Dirofilaria immitis*, the cause of canine heartworms. Microfilariae of *D. immitis* may be noted in blood; however, in the U.S.A., it is important to distinguish the pathogen, *D. immitis*, from the non-pathogen, *Dipetalonema sp.* Positive identification of species depends upon concentration of microfilariae and measurement characteristics. X 100

Figure 13 / 6

Figure 13 / 7

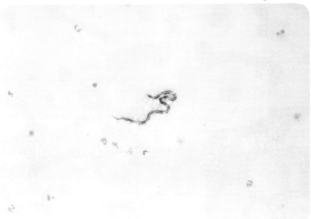

Leukocyte Abnormalities

Inflammation

Following injury the body reacts to eliminate the injurious agent and to repair the damaged tissue. The mechanisms by which the body accomplishes these acts are complex.

Injury alters tissue proteins and causes release of chemical substances that induce increased vascular permeability and dilation. Complement is a key initiating factor in the release of histamine, kinins and prostaglandins that act to increase vascular permeability. Complement (C'3 and C'7) also provides a chemotactic stimulus to neutrophils permitting them access to injured areas. Within a matter of 4-6 hours, neutrophils have accumulated at the injured site. Monocyte migration occurs later. Neutrophils and monocytes are phagocytic and function to eliminate pathogens (bacteria) and to remove dead tissue at the inflammatory site.

Initially, the increased numbers of granulocytes required in inflammation are provided by redistribution within the marginated blood pool and from the storage compartment in the bone marrow. Continued need for neutrophils results in stimulation of the bone marrow with a rise of immature blood neutrophils within 2-3 days. Granulocytes enter the blood stream only to be transported to tissues where they are needed. Hence, granulocytes circulate in the blood for only a few hours never to return. Granulocytes contrast with lymphocytes which may recirculate.

In summary, leukocytes respond to tissue injury; but do not indicate a specific diagnosis.

Functions of Leukocytes

NEUTROPHIL

These are phagocytic cells that function to engulf and destroy bacteria and other particulate matter. The neutrophilic granules (lysosomes) contain hydrolytic and oxidative enzymes that ultimately unite with and kill bacteria.

LYMPHOCYTE

There are two functional types of lymphocytes. One group of lymphocytes, so-called gut associated, are the precursors to plasma cells which produce antibody. The other group are thymic dependent lymphocytes and are associated with cellular immunity. The latter are required for homograph rejection, hypersensitivity reactions and tumor immunity. Increases in total numbers of lymphocytes may indicate lymphosarcoma or recovery from some viral or bacterial infections.

MONOCYTE

The monocyte is a phagocytic leukocyte with granules that contain hydrolytic enzymes. Monocytosis in animals is often associated with diseases in which there is a need to clean the peripheral blood or tissue of debris. A monocytosis may be noted with hemolysis and release of corticosteroids. Monocytes emigrate from blood to tissue forming macrophages. Thus, monocytosis is associated with chronic inflammation in need of tissue macrophages.

EOSINOPHIL

Eosinophilic granules are lysosomes that contain digestive enzymes, notably acid and alkaline phosphatases. Like the neutrophil, the eosinophil is a phagocyte. Eosinophilia is associated with the antigen-antibody complex, especially reactions involving IgE—where the eosinophil is phagocytic destroying these complexes. Eosinophilias are often pronounced where there are antibodies against parasites or following re-exposure to foreign proteins (allergy).

BASOPHIL

Basophils are phagocytic cells that contain hydrolytic enzymes. The granules of the basophil contain heparin, serotonin, and histamine. Histamine and serotonin act to initiate the inflammatory reaction by increasing vascular permeability and attracting leukocytes. Heparin, a potent anticoagulant, is released when there is need for circulating anticoagulant. Basophils are often associated with eosinophilia. Basophilias frequently indicate the need for circulating anticoagulant and may be noted in canine heartworms, equine strongyle infection and allergic respiratory disorders of dogs and cats.

Interpretation of Leukocyte Counts

It is customary to report the total white cell count and give relative percentages of each cell type. The use of the relative percentages or so-called differential count, if considered without taking into account the total count, can result in serious errors. The total number or absolute numbers of cells *must* be calculated for proper interpretation. This calculation can be determined mentally by multiplying the percentage of each cell type by the total count and dividing by 100. As an example, the total leukocyte count in a mature dog is 2,000/cmm with the total lymphocyte percentage of 85. The normal percentage for lymphocytes is 12-30 with the absolute range from 1800-3800/cmm. (APPENDIX II.) This dog has a relative lymphocytosis but a low absolute lymphocyte count ($\frac{85 \times 2000}{100} = 1,700/\text{cmm}$). The relative lymphocytosis draws attention to the possibility of lymphosarcoma but closer inspection reveals that the primary abnormality is an absolute neutropenia. The absolute count suggests another diagnosis.

Causes of Leukocytosis

Leukocytosis is most often the result of absolute increases in numbers of neutrophils. The causes of neutrophilia and leukocytosis may, for diagnostic use, be divided into several categories.

PHYSIOLOGY
Exercise, parturition and emotional upsets may cause a slight leukocytosis. The explanation for this neutrophilia and leukocytosis may be related to the animals enhanced elaboration of corticosteroids.

CORTICOSTEROIDS
Corticosteroids, whether due to elaboration by adrenal cortex or by exogenous treatment, produce a leukocytosis, neutrophilia, lymphopenia, eosinopenia and occasionally a monocytosis.

ACUTE INFECTIONS
Bacterial infections are common causes of neutrophilia and leukocytosis. However, protozoa, fungi and viruses may also produce a neutrophilia.

BLOOD LOSS
A neutrophilia and leukocytosis often accompanies acute hemorrhage or hemolysis.

NEOPLASIA
Rapidly growing malignancies produce neutrophilias. Neoplasia must be considered in the small animal with a persistant leukocytosis and neutrophilia.

NECROSIS
Acute muscle or liver necrosis (by drugs or chemicals) may result in a neutrophilia and monocytosis.

MYELOPROLIFERATIVE DISEASES
Granulocytic leukemia, erythremic myelosis, and erythroleukemia may cause a neutrophilia.

Causes of Leukopenia

Because of the numerical predominance of neutrophils in most animals, a leukopenia is almost always due to a neutropenia. Leukopenia and neutropenia are commonly noted in the following condition.

INFECTIONS
Bacterial—Overwhelming bacterial infections, bacterial endotoxemia, and septicemias commonly cause leukopenias in animals.

Viral—Many specific viral diseases cause leuko-

Leukocyte Abnormalities *cont.*

penia including canine hepatitis, feline panleuko-penia and adenoviral infection of Arabian foals.

Other—A rickettsia, *Ehrlichia canis*, probable cause of Tropical Canine Pancytopenia, produces a leuko-penia, thrombocytopenia and anemia.

IONIZING RADIATION
Radiation therapy is commonly used to treat cancer of animals. An overdose may produce a lymphopenia, neutropenia and also a thrombocytopenia.

DRUGS
Sulfonamides, tetracyclines, possibly chloramphen-icol and cancer therapy drugs can cause leukopenia. There are undoubtedly many chemicals and drugs that produce leukopenia in the occasional animal.

NEOPLASIA
Lymphosarcoma and other myeloproliferative dis-eases can produce leukopenia.

Species Variation in Leukocyte Response

Total numbers and percentages of leukocytes vary in different species of animals.

DOG
Leukocytes response to the inflammation is pro-nounced in the dog. Counts of 30,000 to 40,000/cmm are common and counts between 50,000 to 75,000 are not rare. Band neutrophils are common in high counts but metamyelocytes are rather un-common. Monocytosis may be observed with steroids, chronic infections or hemolysis and a need to clean the blood of debris. Leukopenias are more uncom-mon in the dog than in the cat but may be seen with severe viral or bacterial infections.

CAT
The cat is slightly less responsive to leukocytosis than the dog. However, counts of 30,000 to 40,000/cmm are common while counts between 40,000 to 70,000/cmm are rather uncommon. Band neutro-phils are common and metamyelocytes are not rare. Leukocytosis with an absolute lymphocytosis is re-ported to occur in frightened, excited cats, as well as in some cases of lymphosarcoma. Leukopenia, caused by neutropenia, is very common in the cat.

Some leukopenias are due to panleukopenia virus, infections, myeloproliferative disease and unknown causes. In cats with leukopenias it is common to find giant bands and metamyelocytes with diffuse basophilia of the cytoplasm (toxic neutrophils).

The horse, in comparison, is somewhat less than the cat in its response to inflammation. Leukocyte re-sponse is generally between 15,000-20,000/cmm. Anything above 25,000/cmm is considered to be a marked reaction. Leukocytes are often within the normal range in chronic infections but there may be a neutrophilia. Leukopenias with bands and meta-myelocytes in total counts below 4,000/cmm are occasionally noted with acute septicemias, viral diseases and endotoxic shock.

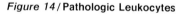

Figure 14 / Pathologic Leukocytes   Figure 14/1

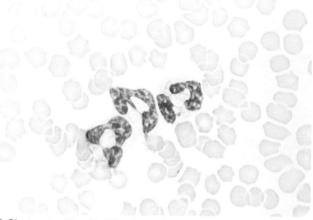

1. A monolobed neutrophil with Dohle bodies (blue cytoplasmic inclusions) as seen in the cat. They represent defective maturation of the neutrophil and are encountered in mild toxemias of the cat.

Figure 14/2

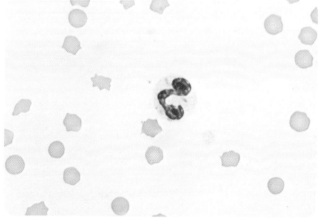

2. Giant neutrophils with diffuse basophilia of the cytoplasm. This is a com-mon manifestation of generalized toxemia in the cat.

Pathologic Leukocytes

3. Hypersegmented neutrophil with 5 nuclear lobes. Increased numbers may be seen as an artifact in old blood, after treatment with corticosteroids (steroids cause neutrophils to circulate for a longer time) in vitamin B12 and folic acid deficiency and in myeloproliferative diseases.

4. Cytoplasmic inclusions in a horse with leukopenia. Specific cause of this equine disease was undetermined.

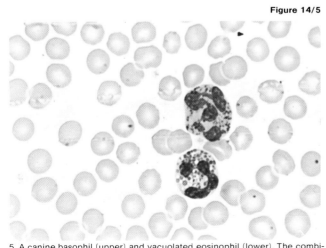

5. A canine basophil (upper) and vacuolated eosinophil (lower). The combination of eosinophilia and basophilia in canine blood suggests heartworms.

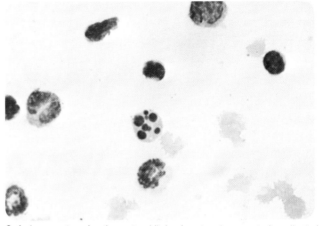

6. A degenerate pyknotic neutrophil. Leukocytes degenerate in collected blood within a few hours. The nucleus of neutrophils first becomes hypersegmented, later the nuclear lobes fragment forming dark pyknotic blobs.

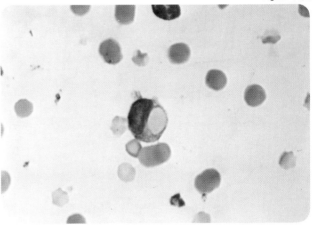

7. Monocyte with phagocytized erythrocyte. Phagocytosis is commonly noted in autoimmune hemolytic anemia.

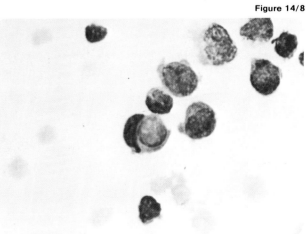

8. A neutrophil with phagocytized magenta-stained nuclear material. Cells having this morphology are called "L.E. cells" and suggest the diagnosis of canine lupus erythematosus.

Thrombocytes

Thrombocytes are released in the bone marrow from the megakaryocyte by the process of cytoplasmic fragmentation. Thrombocytes contribute to hemostasis by providing several coagulation factors (notably Platelet factor 3) as well as forming a platelet plug at small breaks in the blood vessels.

Hemorrhagic diseases of animals are often associated with decreased numbers of thrombocytes. Altered thrombocyte morphology (large, bizarre shaped) are observed in regenerative anemias, myeloproliferative diseases of cats, and other bone marrow disorders.

Thrombocytopenias are noted most often in cats but are only rarely accompanied by serious bleeding. The dog frequently develops severe bleeding problems when the thrombocyte count becomes less than 40,000/cmm. Decreased thrombocytes with bleeding problems are observed in horses.

Thrombocytopenia

The exact mechanisms that cause thrombocytopenias of animals are poorly understood. However, experience has taught us that some diseases may be associated with thrombocytopenia. These diseases include: thrombocytopenia associated with autoimmune hemolytic anemia, lupus erythematosus, overdose of estrogens, consumptive thrombocytopenias caused by tumors (hemangiosarcoma), certain drugs, hypersplenism where reticuloendothelial system destroys thrombocytes, septicemias and myeloproliferative disorders. Recently it has been established that there is antiplatelet activity in the globulin fraction of serum in a majority of dogs diagnosed as idiopathic thrombocytopenic purpura.

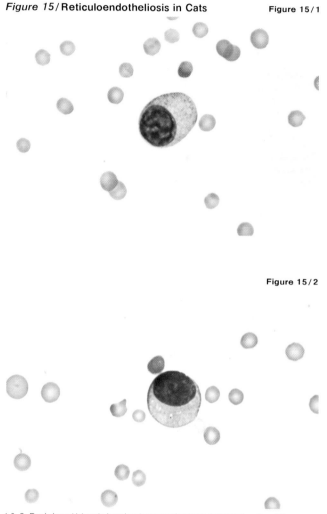

Figure 15 / Reticuloendotheliosis in Cats   Figure 15 / 1

Figure 15 / 2

1 & 2. Peripheral blood showing large reticuloendothelial cells with eccentrically placed nuclei. Cytoplasm is dull blue with prominent pinkish cytoplasmic granules. The cytoplasm in cell 2 contains small vacuoles. PCV was less than 10%, note the absence of polychromasia. X 1000

Myeloproliferative Disease in the Feline

Figure 15/3

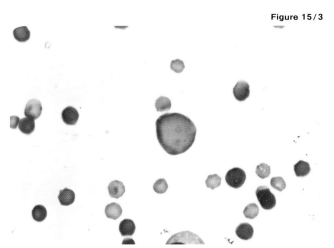

3. Peripheral blood with tremendous anisocytosis yet lacking polychromasia. X 1000

Figure 15/4

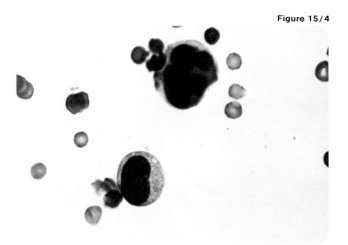

4. Bone marrow with reticuloendothelial cell (lower) and giant megaloblastoid erythrocyte containing 5 nuclei. Megaloblastoid erythrocytes are large, abnormal erythroid cells. They often appear as bizarre rubricytes but occasionally are multinucleated. X 1000

Figure 15/5

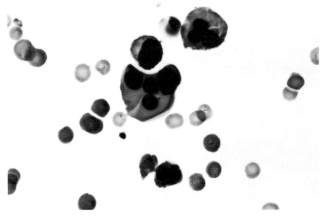

5. Similar to 4, with 2 large megaloblastoid erythrocytes. The presence of megaloblastoid erythrocytes is highly suggestive of myeloproliferative disease. X 1000

Dameshek first hypothesized the concept of a myeloproliferative disorder as a syndrome involving an abnormal proliferation of one or more of the bone marrow cell lines. This disorder encompassed everything from benign hyperplasia to neoplasia of the bone marrow cells. Myeloproliferative disorders are not uncommon in the cat and the proliferation occurs in such a way that various disorders are identified (Table 2). The commonly recognizable cytologic abnormalities in the cat include reticuloendotheliosis, erythremic myelosis, erythroleukemia and granulocytic leukemia.

Common clinical signs associated with myeloproliferative disorder in cats include: anorexia and listlessness of several days to a few weeks duration, weight loss, mucous membrane pallor, elevated temperature, splenomegaly and hepatomegaly with only slight lymph node enlargement. The anemia is generally profound with PCV's as low as 6%. The anemia is non-regenerative in type and therefore reticulocyte count is not elevated. Thrombocytopenia with a few giant cigar forms are commonly noted; however, bleeding problems are rarely observed in the cat.

Blood and Bone Marrow Findings in Cats

RETICULOENDOTHELIOSIS

This myeloproliferative disorder represents an abnormally proliferating undifferentiated cell that has recently been identified as an erythroid precursor cell. Affected cats show a severe anemia without reticulocytosis or significant polychromasia. Thrombocytes are often decreased. The leukocytic count is usually normal but with an average of 20% abnormal, undifferentiated cells (reticuloendothelial cells). The reticuloendothelial cell is large and contains a large often eccentrically placed nucleus that has a chromatin pattern similar to the prorubricyte (Fig. 15). The nucleus often contains a single pale blue nucleolus. Cytoplasm is not abundant but stains dull blue and contains a few pinkish cytoplasmic granules. The bone marrow is replaced with these primitive undifferentiated cells making it difficult to find normal granulocytic and erythroid cells.

ERYTHREMIC MYELOSIS AND ERYTHROLEUKEMIA

The PCVs from cats with either of these 2 forms of myeloproliferative disease is markedly decreased. Anisocytosis is moderate to marked; however, the reticulocyte count is not increased and there are few polychromatophilic erythrocytes. Nucleated erythrocytes are commonly found and if present without a significant reticulocytosis, suggest myeloproliferative disease. The presence of large abnormal nucleated erythroid cells, the so-called "megaloblastoid" erythrocytes, is highly suggestive of myeloproliferative disease. The total leukocyte count is variable, but often leukopenic.

Erythremic myelosis has maturation abnormalities that are limited to the erythrocytic series. Hence, there is a marked proliferation of erythroid cells in the peripheral blood, yet there is an obvious lack of polychromatic erythrocytes (Fig. 16-1). Large, round undifferentiated erythroid precursors with dark royal blue cytoplasm and a large, round nucleus containing a single nucleolus are common in bone marrow (Fig. 16-2). Large megaloblastoid rubricytes may be noted in blood or bone marrow. There is a marked reduction in the granulocytic series of the bone marrow.

Erythroleukemia represents the proliferation of both erythroid and granulocytic cells. The erythroid components are increased in peripheral blood and are similar to those described for erythremic myelosis. The granulocytic component is characterized by the proliferation of immature cells of the granulocyte series. There may be a leukocytosis but more often there is a leukopenia with myeloblasts, progranulocytes and neutrophilic myelocytes comprising the majority of the white cells in circulating blood (Fig. 17). There is a tendency for the proliferating granulocytes to degenerate and to become vacuolated. The bone marrow cytology mirrors the peripheral blood findings except that the proliferation of abnormal cells appears to be more pronounced.

GRANULOCYTIC LEUKEMIA

A leukocytosis with large numbers of immature granulocytes in the circulating blood is only rarely observed in granulocytic leukemia of the cat. The usual findings are advanced anemia without reticulocytosis, leukopenia, and the appearance of an occasional myeloblasts or progranulocyte in peripheral blood (Fig. 18). The bone marrow is hyper-

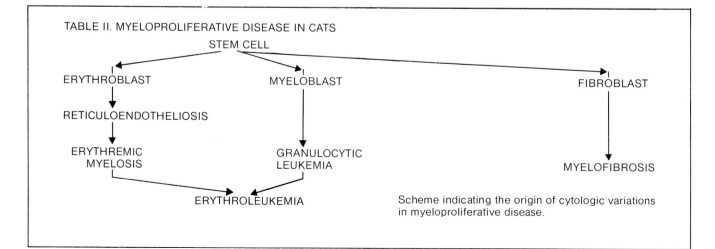

TABLE II. MYELOPROLIFERATIVE DISEASE IN CATS

STEM CELL

ERYTHROBLAST   MYELOBLAST   FIBROBLAST

RETICULOENDOTHELIOSIS

ERYTHREMIC MYELOSIS   GRANULOCYTIC LEUKEMIA   MYELOFIBROSIS

ERYTHROLEUKEMIA

Scheme indicating the origin of cytologic variations in myeloproliferative disease.

cellular with increased numbers of myeloblasts, progranulocytes, myelocytes and mitotic figures (Fig. 18). The granulocytic cells do not appear to mature past the myelocytic stage. Immature erythroid cells are markedly reduced. The increased numbers of progranulocytes with their pinkish cytoplasmic granules classifies the disorder as granulocytic leukemia.

Lymphosarcoma

Lymphosarcoma is a malignant neoplasm commonly observed in dogs and cats. The signs produced are variable and depend greatly on the location of the growing neoplasm. Common signs include lethargy, weight loss, anorexia, fever, diarrhea, dyspnea and enlargement of liver, kidneys, spleen and lymph nodes possibly associated with progressive anemia. Peripheral blood and/or bone marrow may contain abnormal lymphocytes and, are helpful in the diagnosis.

BLOOD AND BONE MARROW FINDINGS

Fifty percent or more of small animals affected with lymphosarcoma have a normal hemogram. Some affected animals have a leukocytosis with a neutrophilia. Others may have a normal to markedly increased leukocyte count with a relative and absolute lymphocytosis. A few atypical, immature lymphocytes confirm the diagnosis of lymphosarcoma (Fig. 20). Anemia, if present, is generally of the nonregenerative type. The bone marrow may occasionally be infiltrated by neoplastic lymphocytes. More than 15% lymphocytes in a hypercellular marrow is suggestive of lymphosarcoma. Care must be taken in the diagnosis of lymphosarcoma from a hypocellular marrow since the disappearance of normal marrow cells causes the normal bone marrow lymphocytes to appear more prominent.

Immature lymphocytes, occurring either in peripheral blood or bone marrow of dogs and cats, are large round cells containing a large often eccentrically placed nucleus with immature, delicate chromatin. Pale blue nucleoli may or may not be noted. The cytoplasm may be vacuolated and is often dark blue and granular with a prominent perinuclear clear zone (Fig. 20). Pseudopod-like cytoplasmic projections may occasionally be observed. One must be able to differentiate these immature lymphocytes from so-called atypical lymphocytes. The most commonly noted atypical lymphocyte in peripheral blood is the immunocyte indicating an immune response while immature lymphocytes suggest lymphosarcoma.

Figure 16/ Erythremic Myelosis in Cats

Figure 16/1

Figure 16/2

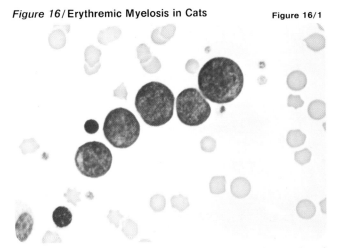

1. Peripheral blood with large, immature erythroid cells. The cytoplasm is dark blue and stippled. Several of these cells contain a single nucleolus. Note the lack of polychromasia. X 1000

2. Bone marrow with immature, erythroid cells. A degenerate reticulum cell is in upper right. X 1000

Figure 17/1

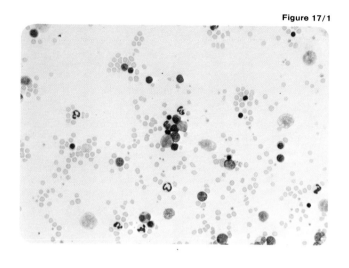

Figure 17 / Erythroleukemia in Felines

1. Peripheral blood with large numbers of nucleated erythrocytes and immature granulocytes. Note the numerous smudged cells that stain pink. X 320

2. Higher magnification of clump of cells in 1, showing clearly the mixture of erythroid and granulocytic cells. Large cell in lower left with nucleolus and few cytoplasmic granules is a progranulocyte, it abuts a rubriblast on the right. X 1000

3. Peripheral blood demonstrating a progranulocyte on top of a rubricyte. X 1000

4. This bone marrow is hypercellular and contains both erythroid and granulocytic cells. There appears to be a piling up of cells with round nuclei. X320

5. Higher magnification of 4, note the 4 progranulocytes in a semicircle, 2 rubricytes, and 1 small undifferentiated cell in upper left. X 1000

Figure 17/2

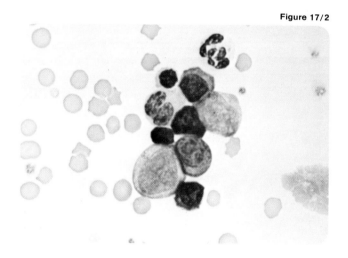

Figure 17/3

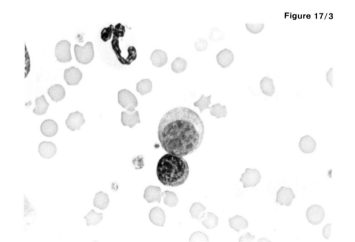

Figure 17/4

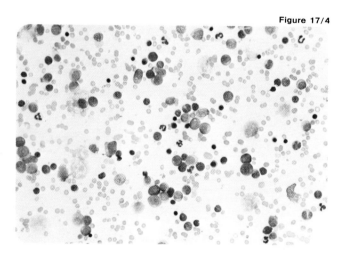

Figure 18/Granulocytic Leukemia

1. Scanning at low magnification revealed a leukopenia (actual count was 2,500/cmm). There were a few large undifferentiated leukocytes, possibly progranulocytes. X 1000

2. The bone marrow revealed large numbers of progranulocytes. Granulocytic cells did not mature past the myelocytic stage. X 1000

3. Same as 2, note the progranulocyte in mitosis. Three lymphocytes are on far left. X 1000

Figure 18/1

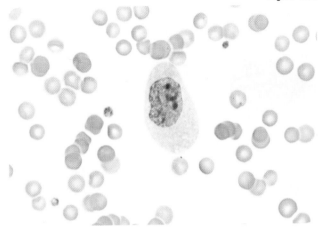

Figure 18/2

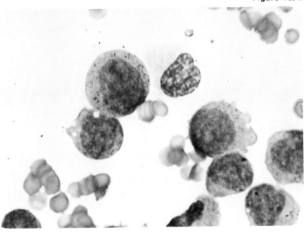

Figure 17/5

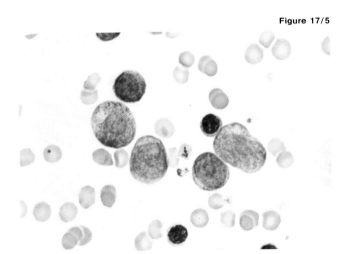

Figure 18/3

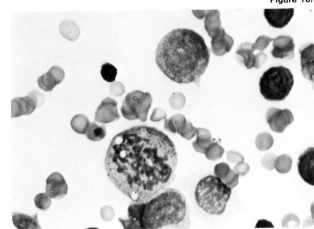

Figure 19/Lymphosarcoma in the Dog

1. Low magnification of peripheral blood showing increased numbers of unidentified mononuclear cells. X 320

2. Higher magnification revealed these cells to be lymphocytes. Two of these lymphocytes are immature, the uppermost cell contains a nucleolus. X 1000

3. Clump of large lymphocytes in blood. An occasional nucleolus is noted. The cytoplasm stains more gray-blue than normal. X 1000

4. Bone marrow packed with neoplastic lymphocytes. Note mitotic figure. X 1000

Figure 19/1

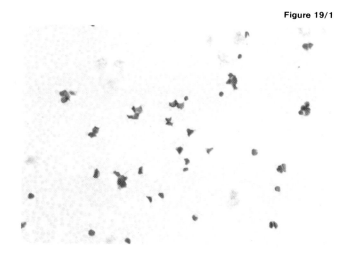

Figure 19/3

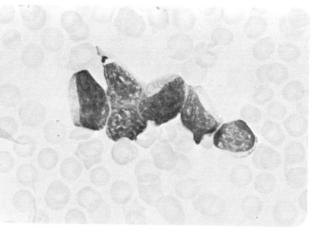

Figure 19/2

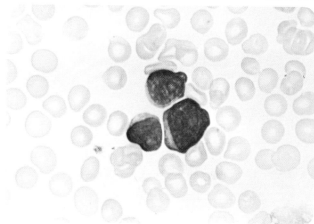

Figure 19/4

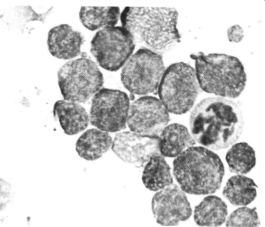

Figure 20/Lymphosarcoma in Cats

1. Peripheral blood with large immature lymphoblast. The nucleus is eccentrically placed with immature nuclear chromatin containing 2 nucleoli. Large pinkish granules seem to overlay the perinuclear clear zone. X 1000

2. Immature lymphocytes similar to 1, except without prominent nucleolus. X 1000

3. Involvement of the bone marrow with neoplastic lymphocytes. X 1000

4. Neoplastic lymphocytes from the thorax of a young cat. These cells are characteristically large with an immature nucleus and basophilic, vacuolated cytoplasm. X 1000

Figure 20/1

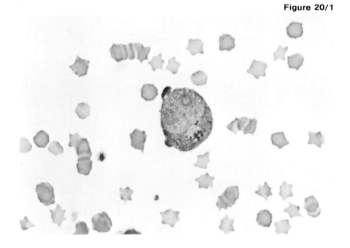

Figure 20/3

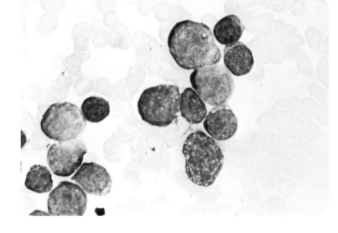

Figure 20/2

Figure 20/4

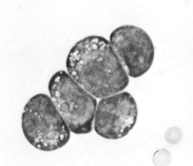

Additional Examples of Leukemia

Figure 21/ **Reticulum Cell Sarcoma Bone Marrow Involvement in a Cat**

1 & 2. Rare reticulum cells observed in peripheral blood. The free nucleus with its prominent, large nucleolus, so characteristic of a disrupted reticulum cell, is seen in 2. The cytoplasm, on the right, is just a blur. X 1000

3. Bone marrow proliferation of reticulum cells. Reticulum cells are large cells with coarse nuclear chromatin. One or 2 distinct, pale blue nucleoli are evident. X 1000

Figure 21/1

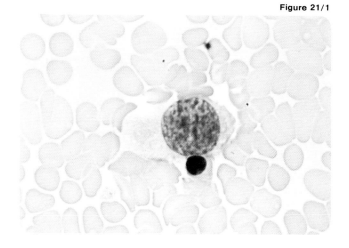

Figure 21/2

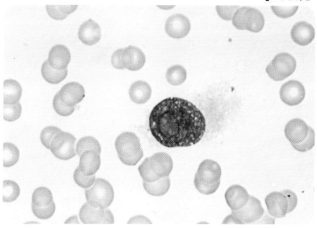

Figure 21/3

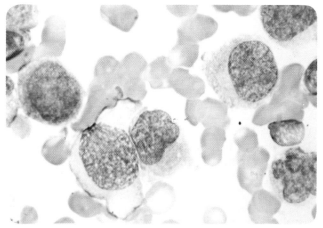

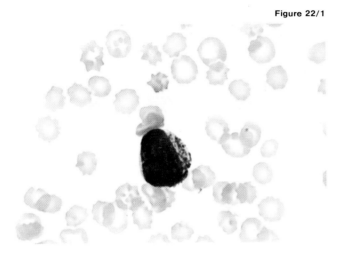

Figure 22/Basophilic Leukemia in a Dog

1 & 2. Examination of peripheral blood revealed a normal leukocyte count (actual count was 11,000/cmm). However, differential count showed 85% to be basophils. These leukocytes were identified as basophils on the basis of the numerous basophilic granules in the cytoplasm. Note that these are basophilic myelocytes and metamyelocytes, not mature basophils. X 1000

3. A majority of the bone marrow cells were basophilic myelocytes. These granules are purple and much more distinct than the granules of the pro-granulocytes. Observe the small mature basophil in the lower middle right. X 1000

Figure 22/2

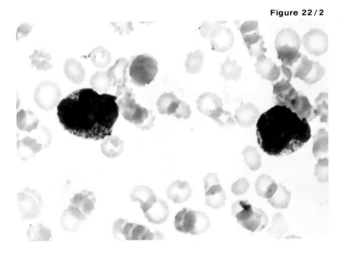

Figure 22/3

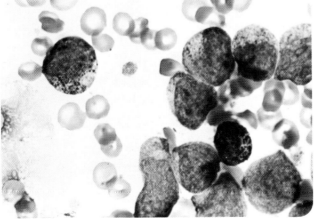

III. Illustrative Cases

The usefulness of blood and bone marrow morphology, as it relates to a specific case, is illustrated in this section. Photographs of actual slides will be used to identify abnormalities in the red blood cells, leukocytes and thrombocytes.

An important part of veterinary practice is the examination of the blood slide. Every slide *must* be examined for abnormalities in numbers and morphology of these 3 cell types. This examination is best performed by first placing oil on the slide and scanning the slide at low magnification (x 100). Using oil at low magnification is to be emphasized since it greatly enhances what is observed. Higher magnification (x 1000) confirms what was suspected at low magnification. Information gained on these 3 cell types is then integrated with the case history, physical examination and other laboratory data. This completely integrated approach often results in a definitive diagnosis as well as suggests specific therapy.

Case 1. *DOG—NORMAL REGENERATIVE RESPONSE IN BLOOD LOSS*

Figure 23/1

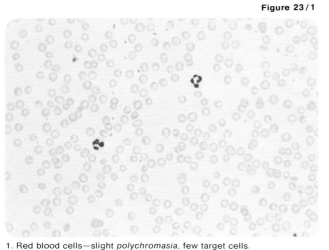

1. Red blood cells—slight *polychromasia*, few target cells.

Leukocytes—normal in number and morphology determined by scanning many fields at low power.

Thrombocytes—normal. X 320

Figure 23/2

2. Confirms that observed at low power. X 1000

Twenty-five percent of the calculated blood volume was removed from a mature dog on day 1, 3, 5, 8 and 9. This blood smear was obtained on day 9 and represents a normal yet rather unremarkable regenerative response. On day 0 the PCV was 40% and had dropped to 24% by day 9. Target cells are commonly observed with polychromasia in regenerative anemias.

Case 1a. *DOG—NORMAL REGENERATIVE RESPONSE IN BLOOD LOSS— RETICULOCYTOSIS*

Figure 24

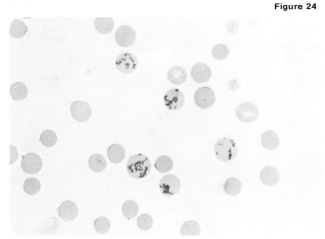

Same as Fig. 23, except blood was first stained with new methylene blue and then counterstained with Wright's stain to demonstrate reticulocytes. Reticulocyte count on day 7 was 7.2%. Leukocytes and thrombocytes are normal in numbers and appearance. X 1000

Case 1b. *DOG—BONE MARROW ERYTHROGENESIS*

Figure 25

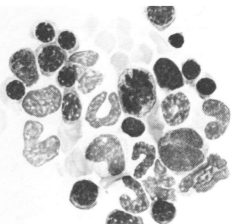

Same as Fig. 23, except this is a bone marrow aspirate demonstrating the modest erythrogenesis that accompanies acute blood loss in the dog. Note the rubricyte in mitosis center and that the nucleated erythrocytes outnumber the granulocytes. X 1000

Case 2. Horse—Acute Blood Loss

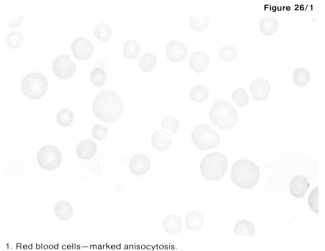

Figure 26/1

1. Red blood cells—marked anisocytosis.
Leukocytes and thrombocytes—normal in numbers and appearance. X 1000

HISTORY
A 7 year old quarter horse gelding was presented because of a cut below the left fetlock joint. The horse had received a wire cut while on pasture 3 or 4 days previous.

LABORATORY FINDINGS
The first day the PCV was 12%, total leukocyte count of 10,600/cmm with a normal differential. Reticulocytes were never increased. Day 14 PCV was 32% and Day 28 PCV was 42%.

TREATMENT
One gallon of blood was given at the time of entry. For the next 4 weeks treatment consisted of antibiotics, good feed and stall rest.

INTERPRETATION
Periodic blood samples demonstrated marked to moderate anisocytosis with occasional Howell-Jolly bodies. The PCV continued to increase and was back in the normal range within a month. The horse is unique in that polychromasia, reticulocytosis, and nucleated red blood cells are not observed as a result of blood loss or hemolysis. With the horse, classification of anemia often depends upon evaluation of the bone marrow.

Case 3. Dog—Chronic Blood Loss—Lice

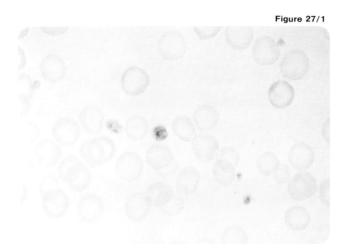

1. Red blood cells—marked hypochromasia (compare with Fig. 23) slight polychromasia, and anisocytosis, an occasional target cell.

Leukocytes and thrombocytes—normal in numbers and appearance. X 1000

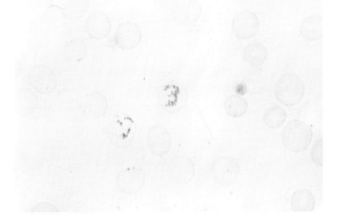

2. Demonstrating increased numbers of erythrocytes with a blue reticulum, reticulocytes. Stained with new methylene blue and counterstained with Wright's stain. X 1000

HISTORY
A 3 year old, male Pekingese was presented because of listlessness for 2-3 weeks. The dog was kept outside and not watched closely.

PHYSICAL EXAMINATION
Mucous membranes appeared pale. Haircoat was poor and there were some reddened areas on abdomen where the dog has been scratching. Closer inspection revealed numerous lice.

LABORATORY FINDINGS
The PCV was 19%, the leukocytic count was 15,400/cmm with a normal differential. There were 2 nucleated RBC/100 WBC and the reticulocyte count was 8.6%. The mean corpuscular volume (MCV) was 60 cubic microns (normal 60-77) and the mean corpuscular hemoglobin concentration (MCHC) was 29% (normal 32-36%).

INTERPRETATION
Small, pale staining (microcytic hypochromic) erythrocytes indicate iron deficiency anemia and in the dog is caused by chronic blood loss. Increased numbers of reticulocytes, and nucleated RBC/100 WBC, along with polychromasia, anisocytosis and poikilocytosis may be noted with chronic blood loss.

ALTERNATE DIAGNOSES
Specific causes of chronic blood loss in the dog include gastrointestinal ulcers, bloody diarrhea, bleeding neoplasma, blood sucking parasites (fleas, lice, ticks) and hookworms.

Case 4. Dog—Autoimmune Hemolytic Anemia (A.I.H.A.)

Figure 28/1

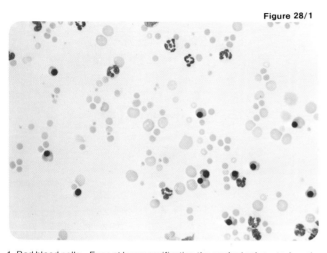

1. Red blood cells—Even at low magnification the marked anisocytosis, poly-chromasia and nucleated erythrocytes are apparent. Small, dense erythro-cytes (spherocytes) are numerous.

Leukocytes—increased in number with a slight increase in bands, a neutro-philia and a monocytosis.

Thrombocytes—normal. X 320

Figure 28/2

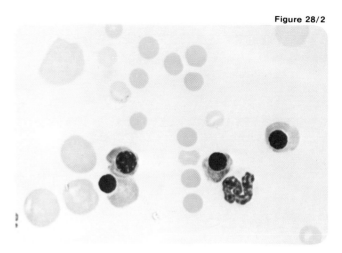

2. Marked anisocytosis, polychromasia with spherocytes, 1 rubricyte, left, and 3 metarubricytes with monolobed neutrophil. X 1000

HISTORY
A 7 month old male St. Bernard was brought to the hospital with the complaint of anorexia for 2 days.

EXAMINATION
The dog was weak and depressed; temperature was 101.1°F. All mucous membranes were pale and yellow.

LABORATORY FINDINGS
Initial hemogram revealed the PCV to be 13%, the WBC count was 65,000/cmm with 85% mature neu-trophils, 4% band, 1% metamyelocyte, 2% lympho-cytes, 7% monocytes, 1% eosinophil, 10% nucleated RBC/100 WBC, and 180,000/cmm thrombocytes. Spherocytes were present and autoagglutination of blood was marked. Coomb's test was markedly positive.

TREATMENT
Injectable prednisolone acetate 20 mg was given t.i.d., along with penicillin-streptomycin b.i.d. and 5% dextrose in Ringers solution.

INTERPRETATION
Spherocytosis, a positive Coomb's antiglobulin test, and spontaneous agglutination of erythrocytes (auto-agglutination) are prominent features of early A.I.H.A. The blood slide shows evidence of an in-tense regenerative response to this anemia with marked reticulocytosis, polychromasia and nucleated RBC's. A leukocytosis between 30,000-70,000/ cmm is not uncommon. There is a neutrophilia with bands and a monocytosis. Increased numbers of monocytes, often observed with hemolytic anemia, are required to remove cellular elements (RBC's) from the blood stream. Erythrophagocytosis may occasionally be observed at the feather edge of the blood slide. Thrombocytopenia may be present in A.I.H.A. but not in this case.

Case 5. Dog—Idiopathic Hemolytic Anemia—Coomb's Negative

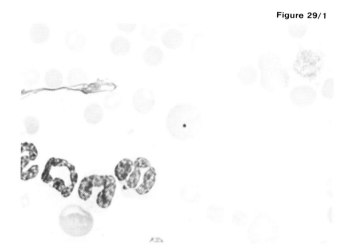

1. Red blood cells—marked anisocytosis, polychromasia, and spherocytosis. Note basophilic erythrocyte with Howell-Jolly body.

Leukocytes—Leukocytosis with neutrophilia, increased bands and monocytosis. Four neutrophils on this slide—1 hypersegmented, 1 band and 2 monolobed.

Thrombocytes—normal in number but many giant forms, upper right. X 1000

2. Another area of slide showing dense, small spherocytes. X 1000

HISTORY
A 2 year old spayed female poodle became listless 4 days previous. A veterinarian gave the dog an injection of antibiotics and vitamins. Corticosteroids were not given. The next day icterus developed, temperature was 104 °F.

PHYSICAL EXAMINATION
The poodle was very depressed, temperature was 101.2°F. Mucous membranes were icteric and appeared pale.

LABORATORY FINDINGS
The initial hemogram revealed a PCV of 11% and total leukocyte count of 75,000/cmm with 75% mature neutrophils, 7% band neutrophils, 1% metamyelocytes, 8% monocytes and 9% lymphocytes. The thrombocyte count was 200,000/cmm. There were 108 nucleated RBCs/100 WBC and the Coomb's test was negative.

TREATMENT
Ten mg of injectable prednisolone acetate was given t.i.d.

INTERPRETATION
Several surveys of autoimmune hemolytic anemia (A.I.H.A.) have been reported. Only those dogs with a positive reaction to the Coomb's test have been diagnosed as A.I.H.A. Many dogs who have had negative reactions to the Coomb's test are identical to dogs who had positive reactions, in regard to laboratory tests (spherocytosis, regenerative anemia). Even though the Coomb's test is negative, some dogs overcome the anemia when treated with corticosteroids. The presence of spherocytes is suggestive of an autoimmune disease mechanism and warrants treatment with steroids. A leukocyte count of 75,000 with a neutrophilia and left shift can be anticipated in association with an intense regenerative erythrocytic response.

Case 6. Dog—Blood Loss Anemia—Hemangiosarcoma

Figure 30/1

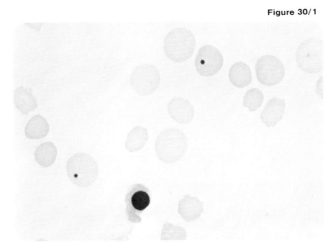

1. Red blood cells—moderate anisocytosis and polychromasia with numerous Howell-Jolly bodies and metarubricytes.

Leukocytes—scanning of several fields revealed normal leukocytes.

Thrombocytes—scanning of feather edge and at higher magnification suggested a thrombocytopenia. X 1000

Figure 30/2

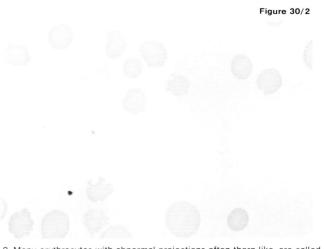

2. Many erythrocytes with abnormal projections often thorn-like, are called acanthocytes. X 1000

HISTORY
An 8 year old spayed female German Shepherd dog was observed by the owner to be weak and slightly depressed. Appetite had been normal. The dog had been on corticosteroids for almost a year for bronchitis.

EXAMINATION
Mucous membranes appeared slightly pale, the abdomen appeared distended, and the liver was enlarged. Temperature was 104.4°F, pulse 180 and respirations were 75/minute.

LABORATORY FINDINGS
The PCV was 34%, a WBC of 14,000/cmm with 85% mature neutrophils, 2% bands, 7% lymphocytes, 3% monocytes and 3% eosinophils. There were 8% nucleated RBC/100 WBC and an occasional spherocyte. Twelve percent of the erythrocytes were reticulocytes. Acanthocytes were numerous (Fig. 30-2). The thrombocyte count was 40,000/cmm.

INTERPRETATION
Hemangiosarcoma involving the liver or spleen should always be considered when an old dog is presented with an abdominal complaint. When blood is lost into a body cavity the bone marrow response is much more intense than if the blood were lost externally. Undoubtedly, this dog was more anemic but the PCV returned towards normal as blood was reabsorbed from the abdominal cavity (autotransfusion). Acanthocytes suggest kidney, liver or splenic disease. Large numbers of nuclear fragments and Howell-Jolly bodies may be observed with splenic neoplasms. A large, hypofunctioning spleen is not capable of removing nuclear remnants. An occasional spherocyte has been observed with hyposplenism. Erythrocytes that remain in the spleen for prolonged periods may become permeable to sodium ions and consequently take the spherical form. Thrombocytopenia, in this case, was likely caused by the consumption of thrombocytes as a result of the activation of the normal coagulation system. This concept of "consumption coagulopathy" and its associated thrombocytopenia is new to the veterinary profession, yet is commonly noted in many types of bleeding diseases.

NECROPSY
The spleen and liver contained many blood-filled soft, red, spongy masses that were determined histologically to be hemangiosarcomas.

Case 7. Dog—Anemia of Renal Disease

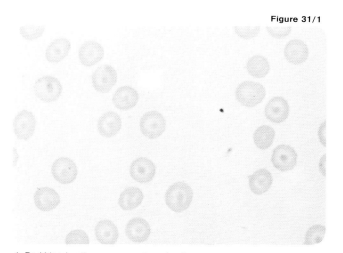

1. Red blood cells—numerous target cells.

Leukocytes—upper range of normal, determined by scanning.

Thrombocytes—normal. X 1000

HISTORY

The 3 year old male Norwegian Elkhound was presented with dyspnea, depression, intermittent fever and not eating or drinking water for one week.

PHYSICAL EXAMINATION

Temperature was 102.8° F, pulse 170, and the dog was panting. The dog appeared humped up in back, pain was severe in upper epigastric region.

LABORATORY FINDINGS

At entry PCV was 27%, WBC was 20,000/cmm with 2% bands, 80% neutrophils, 18% lymphocytes and 4% monocytes. Reticulocytes were less than 1% with only slight anisocytosis and polychromasia. There were large numbers of target cells. The BUN was 138 mg%. Urinalysis revealed a specific gravity of 1.014 with moderate protein; no casts were seen. The remainder of the urinalysis was normal. The PCV continued to drop and 5 days after entry was 16% with less than 1% reticulocytes. The BUN continued to be above 100 mg% and the specific gravity of the urine was fixed (1.010 ± .002). Leptospirosis was not confirmed by serology.

INTERPRETATION

The markedly elevated BUN, fixed specific gravity, and severe anemia without reticulocytosis reflect a poor prognosis. A slight leukocytosis with a neutrophilia and lymphopenia are commonly recognized in dogs with uremia. Increased numbers of target cells may be anticipated in end-stage kidney disease. Lymphosarcoma and chronic infections may also cause nonregenerative anemias in the dog.

RENAL BIOPSY

Basement membranes of glomeruli were thickened with tubules undergoing necrosis and mineralization. There was marked increase in connective tissue in the interstitium. The diagnosis was end-stage kidney disease.

Case 8. Dog—Regenerative Left Shift in Peritonitis

Figure 32/1

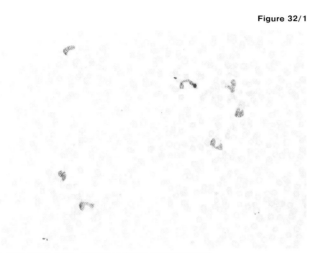

1. Red blood cells—morphologically appear normal.

Leukocytes—slightly increased in numbers, neutrophilia with increased numbers of bands, cytoplasm of neutrophils is noticeably basophilic.

Thrombocytes—normal, clumped at feather edge. X 320

Figure 32/2

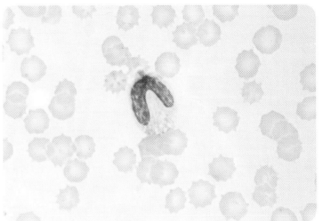

2. Red blood cells are crenated, neutrophilic band with marked basophilia of cytoplasm. X 1000

HISTORY

A 5 year old spayed female German Shorthaired Pointer developed a small lump on the right side of the abdominal wall. This lump ruptured and drained 1 month earlier. Another swelling which developed in the same area disappeared 1 week ago. About the same time the dog became severely ill. Antibiotics did not improve the dog's condition.

PHYSICAL EXAMINATION

Temperature was 102.8°F, the dog was very depressed, showed labored breathing and mucous membranes appeared icteric. The abdomen was painful and distended with fluid.

LABORATORY FINDINGS

The PCV was 28% with slight anisocytosis and polychromasia, reticulocyte count was less than 2%. The plasma was icteric. Leukocyte count was 24,400/cmm with 70% band neutrophils, 10% metamyelocytes, 13% lymphocytes and 7% monocytes. Significant urinalysis findings indicated a specific gravity of 1.014, pH=6, marked bilirubin, and 1-2 granular casts per low power field. The blood urea nitrogen was 70 mg% and the glutamic-pyruvic transaminase (SGPT) was 150 Sigma—Frankel units. Abdominal fluid contained many lysed neutrophils; bacteria were not observed.

INTERPRETATION

Non-regenerative anemias may be caused by chronic infections, chronic renal disease and lymphosarcoma just to mention a few. The non-regenerative anemia, the marked left shift, the presence of toxic, basophilic neutrophils without a significant elevation in leukocytes, suggests a depression of both erythropoiesis and granulopoiesis. It was very difficult to distinguish between monocytes and toxic neutrophils in this case. This severe inflammatory reaction supports an unfavorable prognosis. Blood monocytes travel to tissue and there transform into macrophages; hence, the increased monocytes were required to destroy bacteria and remove tissue debris. The peritonitis caused damage to both kidneys reflected by laboratory findings of high BUN, low urine specific gravity and casts and to the liver reflected by bilirubinuria and high SGPT. *Escherichia coli* and alpha *Streptococcus* were cultured from the peritoneal fluid at necropsy.

Case 9. Dog—Leukocytosis and Non-Regenerative Anemia in Myocarditis

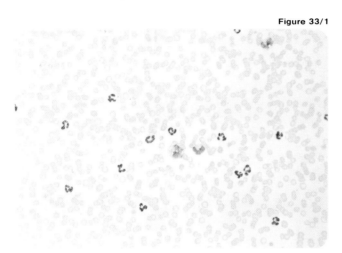

Figure 33/1

1. Red blood cells—morphologically normal.

Leukocytes—leukocytosis with a neutrophilia, a slight left shift and a monocytosis.

Thrombocytes—determined to be normal by finding numerous clumps at feather edge. X 250

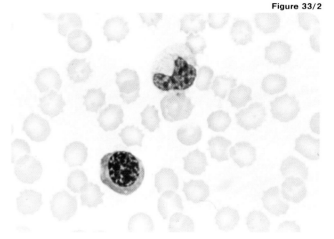

Figure 33/2

2. No polychromasia but note rubricyte and a likely monocyte on the right. X 1000

HISTORY
Three weeks previous a 4 year old male German Shepherd became weak in the rear legs; all paws became swollen. Following this the dog had been depressed and appetite was poor.

PHYSICAL EXAMINATION
Temperature was 103.8 °F. with a pulse rate of 128; the heart sounded normal. There was marked pitting edema of all 4 feet and of the scrotum. The temperature remained above 103 °F. in spite of antibiotic treatment.

LABORATORY FINDINGS
At entry the PCV was 33% but dropped to 19% by the 7th day. On day 1 the WBC count was 31,000/cmm with 3% bands, 78% neutrophils, 8% lymphocytes, 5% monocytes and 6% eosinophils. By day 6 the leukocytic count was 102,000 with 7% bands, 89% neutrophils, 5% lymphocytes, 2% monocytes and 2% eosinophils. Urinalysis revealed a specific gravity of 1.043 with marked proteinuria; no casts were observed. The BUN fluctuated between 10 and 30 mg%.

INTERPRETATION
A persistent elevated temperature in spite of antibiotic therapy, generalized pitting edema, proteinuria and a marked leukocytosis were consistent with bacteremia with embolization of various organs. The chronic infection resulted in severe non-regenerative anemia. Anemia of infection is commonly noted but the mechanism by which the anemia develops is complex and poorly understood. The appearance of nucleated erythrocytes in the absence of polychromasia may be observed in severe inflammation. Endothelial damage that accompanies inflammation may permit these nucleated RBC s to gain entrance to the circulation. The persistent and progressive anemia and leukocytosis suggested an unfavorable prognosis.

NECROPSY
There was marked diffuse infiltration of inflammatory cells in the myocardium. Thrombi and septic emboli were found in the lungs. The renal cortex contained small foci of interstitial fibrosis. The pathologist felt that the myocarditis accounted for the clinical signs of this case.

Case 10. Cat—Degenerative Left Shift in Pyothorax

Figure 34/1

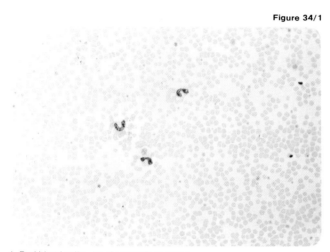

1. Red blood cells—no abnormalities noted.

Leukocytes—within normal range, yet many neutrophilic bands with basophilic cytoplasm. Note the 3 bands.

Thrombocytes—normal. X 320

Figure 34/2

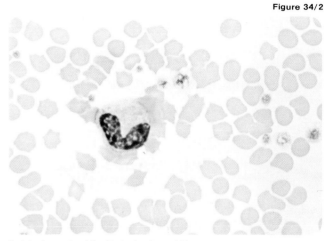

2. A toxic neutrophil with frothy, basophilic cytoplasm; classifying towards the most mature cell type, it would be a neutrophilic band. X 1000

HISTORY
A 1-1/2 year old, castrated male cat was presented because of depression and inappetence for 3 days. The day prior to admittance the cat was unable to stand.

PHYSICAL EXAMINATION
The cat was comatose when admitted. Temperature was 98.4°F., respiration of 80/minute with a pulse of 90/minute. The cat was dyspneic and a fluid line could be percussed.

LABORATORY FINDINGS
The PCV was 43%. The leukocytic count was 10,400/cmm with 3% metamyelocytes, 28% bands, 48% neutrophils, 9% lymphocytes and 12% monocytes.

The neutrophils showed severe toxic changes. Pleural centesis revealed many macrophages and disintegrated neutrophils. Several species of bacteria were engulfed by neutrophils and macrophages.

INTERPRETATION
The bacterial pyothorax caused a toxic depression of granulopoiesis with increased numbers of immature neutrophils with a monocytosis. Monocytes transform into macrophages in the tissue and help to engulf bacteria and debris. Severe toxemias in the cat typically produce a left shift with abnormal morphology of the neutrophil. The severity of the inflammatory disease can often be gauged by the toxic morphology of the neutrophils. Giant neutrophils with frothy, basophilic cytoplasm are characteristic of severe toxicity. Changes in neutrophil morphology towards normal can occur rapidly and suggest remission of disease.

Case 11. Cat—Leukopenia Associated with Subcutaneous Cellulitis

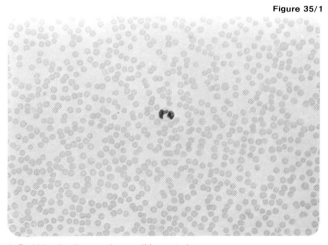

1. Red blood cells—no abnormalities noted.

Leukocytes—marked decrease in numbers, neutrophilic bands were increased and contained basophilic cytoplasm.

Thrombocytes—were present. X 320

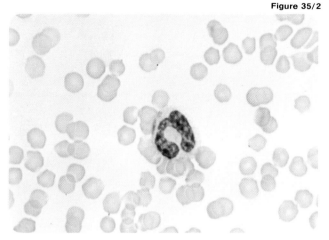

2. Toxic neutrophilic band with a large, coiled nucleus and basophilic cytoplasm. X 1000

HISTORY

A 2 year old male Siamese cat appeared healthy until 5 days ago. The cat stopped eating, was depressed and lay on the heating duct. The cat had no history of vomiting or diarrhea

PHYSICAL EXAMINATION

Temperature was 104 °F.; pulse 170/minute. The mucous membranes were icteric.

LABORATORY FINDINGS

Leukocytic count was 3,600/cmm with 4% metamyelocytes, 22% band neutrophils, 66% neutrophils and 8% lymphocytes. The neutrophils were large with basophilic, foamy cytoplasm. The PCV was 32%. The urinalysis revealed a specific gravity of 1.034 with a large amount of bilirubin present; the remainder of the urinalysis was normal. The BUN was 80 mg% and the SGPT was 200 with the normal being less than 50 Sigma—Frankel units. Bone marrow was hypocellular with both erythroid and granulocytic cells decreased. The granulocytic cells were generally larger and contained basophilic, vacuolated cytoplasm. Neutrophilic metamyelocytes and bands were the predominant cell type in the marrow.

INTERPRETATION

A leukopenia with a pronounced left shift suggests that bone marrow is incapable of producing mature neutrophils; this was confirmed by bone marrow aspiration. Toxic as well as increased numbers of immature neutrophils justify a very poor prognosis. A slightly elevated SGPT indicates mild liver disease while the elevated BUN was likely caused by poor perfusion of the kidneys.

NECROPSY

The subcutis contained some yellowish, cloudy fluid with large numbers of neutrophils. Histologically, the morphologic diagnosis was necrotizing cellulitis. The liver had areas of centrolobular necrosis felt to be secondary to septicemia and toxemia.

Case 12. Cat—Hemolytic Anemia and Leukopenia Associated with Methylene Blue Toxicity

Figure 36/1

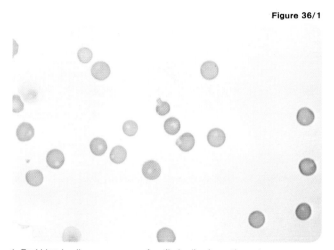

1. Red blood cells—numerous refractile bodies in erythrocytes.
Leukocytes—scanning at low magnification revealed decreased numbers.
Thrombocytes—normal. X 1000

Figure 36/2

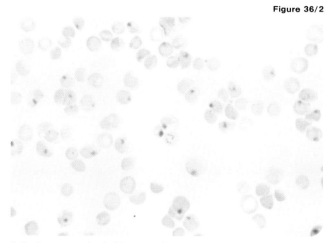

2. Erythrocytes stained with new methylene blue, note numerous blue Heinz bodies. X 1000

HISTORY

A 4 year old male castrated Siamese developed urethral obstruction 1 month ago. Catheterization relieved the obstruction. Two weeks later the cat re-obstructed; catheterization was again successful. The cat had been treated for 1 month with Chloramphenicol and Urisept (methylene blue 5.4 mg) 1 tablet 3 times a day. The cat had been vomiting once or twice a day for the last 2 weeks.

PHYSICAL EXAMINATION

Temperature was 99 °F. with a heart rate of 200/minute. The cat was depressed and the mucous membranes were pale. Green urine was expressed through a patent urethra. Urisept tablets were discontinued.

LABORATORY FINDINGS

PCV was 11%, leukocytic count was 3,600/cmm with 70% neutrophils, 27% lymphocytes, 2% monocytes and 1% eosinophils. Many erythrocytes contained large Heinz bodies when stained with new methylene blue. No reticulocytes or nucleated RBC's were observed. The bone marrow was hypoplastic in regards to both nucleated erythrocytes and granulocytes. Heinz bodies were prominent in marrow erythrocytes. Ringers Lactate and 50 ml of whole blood were given intravenously. Six days after transfusion rubriblasts and prorubricytes were identified in bone marrow. By the 9th day there were 8.6% reticulocytes with 100 nucleated RBC/100 WBC, the leukocytic count was 15,400 with 1% metamyelocyte, 3% bands, 60% neutrophils, 32% lymphocytes, 3% monocytes and 1% eosinophil.

INTERPRETATION

Urinary antiseptic drugs that contain methylene blue can cause hemolytic anemia in the cat. The anemia is characterized by inclusion bodies (Heinz or erythrocyte-refractile bodies) within many erythrocytes. Supravital stains, such as new methylene blue, clearly demonstrate the presence of these refractile bodies. In this particular cat the methylene blue resulted in severe depression of erythropoiesis and granulopoiesis. Six days after discontinuing the drug, the bone marrow was producing erythrocytes and granulocytes.

The use of methylene blue in cats should be discontinued.

Case 13. Horse—Leukopenia Associated with Salmonellosis

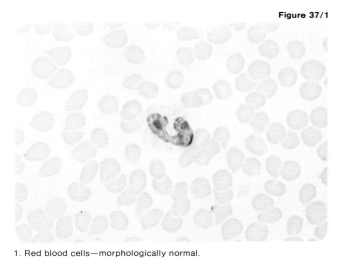

1. Red blood cells—morphologically normal.

Leukocytes—scanning suggested a possible leukopenia. Numerous bands and occasional metamyelocytes were encountered. They were toxic with basophilic, vacuolated cytoplasm. Note toxic band.

Thrombocytes—normal. X 1000

2. Two metamyelocytes with basophilic, vacuolated cytoplasm. X 1000

HISTORY
A 10 year old quarter horse mare was severely stressed by a 1300 mile trailer ride within a 24 hour period. She was depressed on arrival and went completely off feed 3 days later. Antibiotics did not prevent the development of severe diarrhea 2 days later. Temperature was 103 °F.

PHYSICAL EXAMINATION
Temperature was 103.8°F., and heart rate 84/minute. The mare was dehydrated, depressed and had watery diarrhea.

LABORATORY FINDINGS
PCV was 53%, total plasma protein was 8.5 gm%, WBC count was 5,000/cmm with 10% metamyelocytes, 40% bands, 12% neutrophils, 37% lymphocytes and 1% monocyte. The cytoplasm of the neutrophils was foamy and basophilic. *Salmonella typhimurium* type B was isolated by fecal culture.

INTERPRETATION
The elevated PCV and plasma protein signify moderate dehydration. The leukopenia, marked left shift and toxic neutrophils indicated a severe disease process with a grave prognosis. Leukopenia with toxic neutrophils is a common sequela to endotoxemia in the horse. The presence of salmonella organisms along with the necropsy findings of acute colitis support the diagnosis of Salmonellosis.

Case 14. Dog—Steroid Responsive Thrombocytopenia

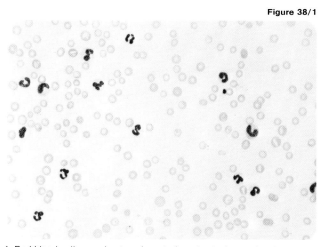

Figure 38/1

1. Red blood cells—moderate anisocytosis and polychromasia, slight hypochromasia and a few target cells.

Leukocytes— a leukocytosis, neutrophilia with a few bands and a monocytosis.

Thrombocytes—no clumps observed at feather edge. X 320

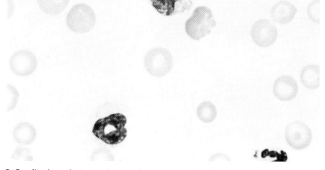

Figure 38/2

2. Confirming what was observed at low magnification, note band, monocyte and segmented neutrophil. X 1000

HISTORY
A five year old male Collie had excessive tartar on teeth with ulceration of gums and oral mucosa. Dentistry was followed by persistent bleeding. The muzzle became swollen and epistaxis developed the day following surgery.

PHYSICAL EXAMINATION
Depression was pronounced; mucous membranes were pale. Blood was oozing from gums and there were soft tissue swellings over both hock joints and over the muzzle.

LABORATORY FINDINGS
The leukocyte count was 103,000/cmm with 3% metamyelocytes, 8% bands, 81% neutrophils, 2% lymphocytes, 5% monocytes, 1% eosinophil and 6% nucleated RBC/100 WBC. The PCV was 14% and the BUN was 20 mg%. Thrombocytes were less than 10,000/cmm; Coomb's test and L.E. cell preparations were negative.

TREATMENT
Injectable prednisolone (10 mg twice daily) and penicillin and streptomycin were started on the first day.

FOLLOW-UP LAB RESULTS
The thrombocyte count one day following steroid treatment was 31,000/cmm on day 2 the count was 77,000/cmm and on day 5 the count was 150,000/cmm. The leukocyte count had dropped to 48,000/cmm by the 5th day.

INTERPRETATION
The cause of thrombocytopenia was not apparent. There was a marked regenerative anemia which is to be anticipated in massive hemorrhage. A leukocytosis with a left shift is expected, although excessive in this case, with a regenerative anemia. Monocytes were needed to remove erythrocytes in tissues. Treatment of steroids ushered in the reappearance of thrombocytes along with the disappearance of hemorrhage.

IV. Appendix I.
Staining of Blood and Bone Marrow — Wright's Stain

Material Purchased From:

> Harleco
> Hartman-Leddon Company
> 60th & Woodland Avenue
> Philadelphia, Pennsylvania
> 19143

Wright's Stain: #508 Wright Blood Stain
> Package 10 units, each unit
> containing 0.5 gm

> Dissolve 1 unit (0.5 gm) in 300 ml of absolute methyl alcohol. Make up 1 to 2 gallons of Wright's stain at a time so it can age. The longer the stain ages the better its staining properties. Place about 1 to 2 mls of 10% formalin in each gallon of stain to prevent bacteria from growing.

Wright's Buffer: #4022 Buffer Salt Mixture, pH 6.8

> Dissolve 1 gm of buffer in 1000 ml of neutral distilled water. Distilled water is often acid, make it neutral by adding enough 1% potassium bicarbonate until pH paper indicated neu-trality. New buffer has to be made up every few days. Keep buffer in the refrigerator.

PROCEDURE:

The staining rack technique is recommended. The staining and buffering time must be determined for each batch of stain.

Peripheral Blood

1. Flood slide with stain for 3 minutes.
2. Add equal amounts of buffer to slide being careful not to wash off stain; blow gently, mixing stain and buffer. A greenish sheen will develop on the slide.
3. After 5-10 minutes wash slide thoroughly with tap water. Wipe off back of slide with a tissue or gauze and air dry.

Bone Marrow

Stain as peripheral blood slide except allow the stain and buffer mixture to remain on slide for 10-20 minutes before washing.

Appendix II.
Normal Blood Values for Dogs

	Male			Female		
Blood Test	Puppy (Birth to 12 mos.)	Adult (1 to 7 years)	Geriatric (7 years or older)	Puppy (Birth to 12 mos.)	Adult (1 to 7 years)	Geriatric (7 years or older)
Hemoglobin (gm/100ml)	6.9-16.5	12.7-16.3	14.7-21.2	6.4-18.9	11.5-17.9	11.0-22.5
Hematocrit (%)	22.0-45.0	35.2-52.8	44.2-62.8	25.8-55.2	34.8-52.4	35.8-67.0
Red Blood Cells (mil.)	2.99-8.52	5.26-6.57	3.33-7.76	2.76-8.42	5.13-8.6	3.34-9.19
White Blood Cells (10^3)	9.9-27.7	8.3-19.5	7.9-35.3	8.8-26.8	7.5-17.5	5.2-34.0
Neutrophils (%)	63-73	65-73	55-80	64-74	58-76	40-80
Lymphocytes (%)	18-30	9-26	15-40	13-28	11-29	13-45
Monocytes (%)	1-10	2-10	0-4	1-10	0-10	0-4
Eosinophils (%)	2-11	1-8	1-11	1-9	1-10	0-19
Basophils	rare	rare	rare	rare	rare	rare
Total Protein (gm/100ml)	3.90-5.90	4.90-9.60	5.5-7.3	4.00-6.40	5.50-7.80	4.7-7.5

Appendix II.
Normal Blood Values for Cats

	Male			Female		
Blood Test	Kitten (Birth to 12 mos.)	Adult (1 to 5 years)	Geriatric (6 years or older)	Kitten (Birth to 12 mos.)	Adult (1 to 5 years)	Geriatric (6 years or older)
Hemoglobin (gm/100ml)	6.0-12.9	8.9-17.0	9.0-14.5	6.0-15.0	7.9-15.5	7.5-13.7
Hematocrit (%)	24.0-37.5	26.9-48.2	28.0-43.8	23.0-46.8	25.3-37.5	22.5-40.5
Red Blood Cells (10^3)	5.43-10.22	4.48-10.27	5.26-8.89	4.46-11.34	4.45-9.42	4.10-7.38
White Blood Cells (10^3)	7.8-25.0	9.1-28.2	6.4-30.4	11.0-26.9	13.7-23.7	5.2-30.1
Neutrophils (%)	16-75	37-92	33-75	51-83	42-93	25-89
Lymphocytes (%)	10-81	7-48	16-54	8-37	12-58	9-63
Monocytes (%)	1-5	1-5	0-2	0-7	0-5	0-4
Eosinophils (%)	2-21	1-22	1-15	0-15	0-13	0-15
Basophils	rare	rare	rare	rare	rare	rare
Total Protein (gm/100ml)	4.3-10.0	6.8-10.0	6.2-8.5	4.8-9.1	6.6-8.9	6.0-9

Appendix III.
Normal Blood Values for Dog and Cat*

BLOOD TEST	DOG	CAT
M.C.V. (u^3)	60-77	40-55
M.C.H.C. %	32-36	30-36
Bone Marrow M:E Ratio	0.75-2.5	0.60-3.9

*From Schalm 1965.

Appendix IV.
Normal Blood Values for the Horse*

BLOOD TEST	HORSE
Hematocrit (%)	32-52
Hemoglobin (Gms %)	11-19
R.B.C. (10^6)	6.7-13
Total Protein	5.3-7.6
W.B.C. (10^3)	5.5-12.5
Differential	% (Absolute)
Bands	0-2 (0-100)
Segs	30-65 (2700-6700)
Lymphocytes	25-70 (1500-5500)
Monocytes	0-7 (0-800)
Eosinophils	0-11 (0-925)
Basophils	0-3 (0-170)
M.C.V. (u^3)	34-58
M.C.H.C. %	30-36
Bone Marrow M:E Ratio	0.94-3.76

*From Schalm 1965.

Selected References

1. 1949, Condensation of the first two reports of the committee for clarification of the nomenclature of cells & diseases of the blood and blood-forming organs. Blood, 4:89.

2. Dameshek, W., 1951, Some speculation on the myeloproliferative syndrome. Blood, 6:372.

3. David, G. B. and B. S. Williamson 1971. Amplitude—contrast microscopy in histochemistry. Histochemie, 27:1.

4. De Robertis, E. D., W. W. Nowinski and F. A. Saez 1970. Cell Biology, 5th ed. W. B. Saunders Co., Philadelphia, Pa.

5. Diggs, L. W., D. Sturm and A. Bell 1970. The Morphology of Human Blood Cells, Abbott Labboratories, North Chicago, Ill.

6. Good, R. A. and D. W. Fisher 1971. Immunobiology. Sinauer Associates, Inc. Stamford, Conn.

7. Greenwalt, T. J. and G. A. Jamieson 1970. Formation & Destruction of Blood Cells. J. B. Lippincott, Co. Philadelphia, Pa.

8. Jensen, K. G. and S. A. Killman 1970. Aspects of inflammation I & II. Series Haematologica.

9. Jensen, K. G. and S. A. Killman 1968. Leukocytes: eosinophils, basophils, biochemistry. Series Haematologica, 1:3.

10. La Via, M. F. and R. B. Hill 1971. Principles of Pathobiology. 1st ed., Oxford University Press, Inc., New York.

11. Lewis, R. W., R. S. Schwartz and C. E. Gilmore 1965. Autoimmune diseases in domestic animals. Ann. N. Y. Acad. Sci., 124:178.

12. Miale, J. B. 1972. Laboratory Medicine Hematology. 4th ed., Chapter 2. The reticuloendothelial system II, Lymphocytes & the immunocyte complex. C. V. Mosby Co., St. Louis, Mo.

13. Perman, V. and J. B. Stevens 1971. Leukocyte responses in health & disease. Proc AAHA, 38th annual meeting, p. 420.

14. Pitney, W. R. 1971. Disseminated intravascular coagulation. Seminars in Hematology, 8:65.

15. Schalm, O. W. 1971. Cytology of some myeloproliferative disorders of cats. Feline Practice. 1:23.

16. Schalm, O. W. 1969. Hematologic characteristics of autoimmune hemolytic anemia in the dog. Calif. Vet. 23:19.

17. Schalm, O. W. 1972. Interpretations in feline bone marrow cytology. J. Amer. Vet. Med. Ass. 161:1418.

18. Schalm, O. W. 1971. The blood platelets (thrombocytes): I. Production & function. Calif. Vet. 25:6.

19. Schalm, O. W. 1971. The blood platelets (thrombocytes): II. The thrombocytopathics. Calif. Vet. 25:6.

20. Schalm, O. W. 1965. Veterinary Hematology. 2nd. ed., Lea & Febiger, Philadelphia, Pa.

21. Schechter, R. D., O. W. Schalm and J. J. Kaneko 1973. Heinz body hemolytic anemia associated with the use of urinary antiseptics containing methylene blue in the cat. J. Amer. Vet. Med. Ass. 162:37.

22. Wilkins, R. J., A. I. Hurvitz and J. Dodds-Laffin 1973. Immunologically mediated thrombocytopenia in the dog. J. Amer. Vet. Med. Ass. 163:277.

Glossary of Terms

ACANTHOCYTES—Erythrocytes with abnormal blunt projections.

ANISOCYTOSIS—Variation in size of erythrocytes.

ATYPICAL—Not normal, not usual.

AUTOAGGLUTINATION—Spontaneous clumping or agglutination of erythrocytes in drawn blood.

AUTOIMMUNE DISEASES—An immunologic disorder whereby the body destroys part of itself; with erythrocytes an antibody attaches to its membrane causing early destruction by the body.

AZUROPHILIC GRANULES—Cytoplasmic granules that generally stain pink with Wright's stain, often noted in lymphocytes and monocytes.

BAND CELL—A leukocyte in which the nucleus has smooth, parallel sides with only slight indentation.

BASOPHILIC—Capability of staining various intensities of blue with Wright's stain.

BASOPHILS—Granulocytes containing purplish to blue-black (canine) or lavender (feline) cytoplasmic granules and slightly lobulated nuclei.

CHROMATIN—The cel nucleus which readily stains and is composed of desoxyribose nucleic acid (DNA).

COOMB'S TEST—An erythrocyte agglutination test which when positive indicates the presence of globulin autoantibodies on erythrocyte surfaces.

CRENATION—The margins of erythrocytes appearing as sharp points.

DEOXYRIBONUCLEIC ACID (DNA)—The nucleic acid present in the nucleus that controls the amino acid sequence of proteins.

DÖHLE BODIES—Discrete blue staining oval bodies that are often found in cat neutrophils; may represent toxemic effect of disease.

EOSINOPHILIC—Capable of staining various degrees of red with Wright's stain.

EOSINOPHILS—Granulocytes containing prominent granules that stain red with Wright's stain.

ERYTHREMIC MYELOSIS—Abnormal proliferation of erythrocytic cells in peripheral blood and bone marrow.

ERYTHROCYTE REFRACTILE BODIES (ER BODIES)—Same as Heinz bodies.

ERYTHROCYTES—Mature red blood cells.

ERYTHROID CELLS—Cells of the erythrocytic series.

ERYTHROLEUKEMIA—Neoplastic proliferation simultaneously of erythroid and granulocytic cells in blood and bone marrow.

ERYTHROPHAGOCYTOSIS—The condition of having erythrocytes engulfed.

FIXED TISSUE CELLS — Immobile, large cells in bone marrow.

GOLGI APPARATUS—A complex of cytoplasmic membranes and vesicles which is concentrated into a light zone adjacent to the nucleus. Concerned with synthesis of carbohydrates and packaging of secretions.

GRANULOCYTES—Cells that develop in the bone marrow and contain readily identifiable cytoplasmic granules. Neutrophils, eosinophils and basophils are granulocytes.

HEINZ BODIES—Refractile inclusions of denatured hemoglobin often noted in cat erythrocytes. These inclusions may cause bulging of erythrocytes. With new methylene blue stain the bodies are blue-black.

HOWELL-JOLLY BODIES—Retained round nuclear fragments within erythrocytes.

HYPOCHROMASIA—Decreased hemoglobin in erythrocytes causing lighter color when stained.

HYPERSEGMENTED NEUTROPHIL—Neutrophils that contain more than four distinct nuclear lobes.

IMMATURE CELLS—Cells not fully developed.

IMMUNOCYTES (SYNONYM—REACTIVE LYMPHOCYTE)—Cells formed from lymphocytes when antigen is present; cells likely synthesizing immune globulins.

LARGE LYMPHOCYTES—Lymphocytes about two to three times as large as small lymphocytes.

LEUKEMIA—A neoplastic disease characterized by proliferation of the cells of bone marrow or peripheral blood.

LYSOSOMES—Appear as cytoplasmic granules within some cells, contain digestive enzymes.

MEGAKARYOCYTES—Giant cells with lobulated nucelei, occurring in bone marrow, and presumed to generate blood platelets.

METARUBRICYTES—Immature red blood cells in a stage of development where the nucleus appears as a dark blue homogeneous mass without any distinct chromatin structure.

MONOCYTES—Large leukocytes with oval or indented, pale nuclei, having more cytoplasm than lymphocytes, the cytoplasm is often vacuolated.

MONOLOBED NEUTROPHILS—Most commonly occurring animal granulocyte, in development stage between band neutrophils and segmented neutrophils.

MYELOBLASTS—Immature cells from "stem cells" developing to progranulocytes.

MYELOCYTES—Immature cells developed from progranulocytes; the granules can be differentiated into neutrophilic, eosinophilic or basophilic according to the staining properties of their granules.

MYELOPROLIFERATIVE DISEASES—Diseases associated with abnormal proliferation of blood or bone marrow cells.

NEUTROPHILS—Mature white blood cells which contain small cytoplasmic granules that are lysosomes. They are phagocytic cells that function to engulf and destroy bacteria and other particulate matter.

NON-REGENERATIVE ANEMIA—The increase in red cell precursors in blood and bone marrow is less than expected for the degree of anemia.

OSTEOBLASTS—Bone-forming cells rarely noted on aspiration of bone marrow.

OSTEOCLASTS—Large multi-nucleated cells functioning in the absorption and removal of bone tissue.

PATHOLOGIC CYTOLOGY—Cell morphology associated with diseases.

PHAGOCYTOSIS—Ingestion and digestion by cells.

PLASMA CELLS—Ovoid cells with eccentrically placed nuclei which produce antibodies.

PLATELETS—Thrombocytes, or irregularly-shaped cells containing granules but having no definable nuclei.

POIKILOCYTOSIS—The presence of irregularly shaped red blood cells in peripheral blood.

POLYCHROMASIA—The tendency of red blood cells to stain basophilic; young erythrocytic cells. Synonym —basophilia.

PROGRANULOCYTES—Developmental cell stages between myeloblasts and myelocytes.

PROMEGAKARYOCYTES—Cells in stage of development from megakaryoblasts to megakaryocytes.

PRORUBRICYTES—Developing cells in the stage from rubriblasts to rubricytes.

REGENERATIVE ANEMIA—There is evidence of increased red blood cell production in blood and bone marrow (polychromasia, reticulocytosis).

RETICULOCYTES—Young, large erythrocytes that contains a blue reticulum when stained with new methylene blue.

RETICULOCYTOSIS—Term applied when the reticulocytes are increased above normal.

RETICULOENDOTHELOSIS—An abnormal proliferation of an early erythroid precursor cell.

RETICULUM CELLS—Large, fragile bone marrow cells identified by their coarse, linear nuclear chromatin and prominent nucleoli.

RIBONUCLEIC ACID (RNA)—The nucleic acid that is synthesized in the nucleus but acts in the cytoplasm to form proteins.

ROULEAU (ROULEAUX, PLURAL)—Red blood cells affixed in groups resembling stacks of coins.

RUBRIBLASTS—Immature cells in stage of development from stem cells to prorubricytes.

RUBRICYTES—Immature blood cells in stage of development to metarubricytes.

SEGMENTED NEUTROPHIL—A cell containing specific neutrophilic granules where the lobes of the nucleus are connected by fine nuclear filaments.

SMALL LYMPHOCYTES—Believed to be the same in the bone marrow as "stem cells"; in peripheral blood slightly larger than erythrocytes.

SPHEROCYTES—Dense spherical canine erythrocytes that appear to be smaller than normal erythrocytes.

STELLATE—Star-shaped.

TARGET CELLS—Irregularly shaped erythrocytes with the appearance of a target.

THROMBOCYTES—Same as platelets.

THROMBOCYTOPENIAS—Conditions in which abnormally small numbers of platelets are circulating in the blood.

Index

(Prepared by Doris B. Marshall)